The Handbook of Curanderismo:

A Practical Guide to the Cleansing Rites of Mesoamerican Shamans and Curanderos

Juan Espinoza

Warning-Disclaimer

The purpose of this book is to educate and entertain. The author or
publisher does not guarantee that anyone following the techniques,
suggestions, tips, ideas, or strategies will become successful. The
author and publisher shall have neither liability or responsibility to
anyone with respect to any loss or damage cause, or alleged to be
cause, directly or indirectly by the information contained in this
book.

IMPORTANT WARNING!!!

The different remedies cited here come from the popular and
folkloric traditions and the author's great fondness for collecting
medicinal recipes by rummaging here and there. This does not mean,
far from it, that it is advisable to put them all into practice, although
the efficacy of some of them is sufficiently proven. We warn with
this that if anyone wants to try any of the remedies here exposed, in
himself or other people, he will do it under his exclusive
responsibility and with all its consequences.

All that the healer claims to cure

IMPORTANT WARNING!!!

TABLE OF CONTENTS

INTRODUCTION

Let no one is deceived when reading this book. The reader is not before a work of a practical or didactic type, although everything that is said in it has been used, in its time, as a curative remedy by one or another people. But the reader is, however, before an informative synthesis that intends to satisfy an anthropological curiosity that is less well known than it is believed. Everything that appears in the book is the result of the investigations of the most diverse and qualified folklorists and the contrast that, through very diverse essays and manuals, some of the great modernity have carried out in their moment prestigious doctors.

There are many who confuse "folk medicine" with "natural medicine". Many, especially in recent years, have shown great interest in the subject. And some continue to identify "folk medicine" with "home remedies". To tell the truth, since to err is human and medicine is human in its broadest concept, the rightness, in this case, is not exclusive to anyone. Only one thing is certain: that the success of a given curative practice, whether it is considered scientific or not, only serves the individual insofar as it remedies an ailment. Or, to put it another way: all medicine, as long as it cures, is good.

To understand what has come to be called "folk medicine", we must place ourselves in an indeterminate but very remote period of history. But it cannot be overlooked that the existential evolution of some cultures, with respect to others, has not always run chronologically speaking, evenly. For example, as historical researchers are confirming, while already in the Egyptian empire, the advances in medicine were amazing and were applied in a scientific way, all of what was later to become Europe had yet to shake off that period that we know as prehistory, that is, a long period of material and spiritual backwardness, if observed from a comparative point of view. In other words, while certain peoples were very advanced, others still lived in a primitive way, as is still the case today with certain tribes and ethnic groups wrongly called savages.

Well, suppose we put ourselves in the place of those remote cultures. In that case, we will find an immaculate geographical environment, that is to say, unaltered by introducing artificial elements. A land that the various contemporary romantic movements have wanted to intuit as paradisiacal, but which must have been quite the opposite if we analyze the matter coldly. In that environment man was, so to speak, at the mercy of the elements. Faced with adversity, he had to improvise solutions inspired by his own and still scarce knowledge and look for new ones if the result did not satisfy him. Partly by the instinct of conservation, partly thanks to chance, he discovered a series of practical methods that, besides helping him to survive, made his existence more comfortable. He learned to make utensils for domestic use and weapons that made hunting and warfare easier, discovering at the same time the way to transform for his benefit the raw elements that the earth offered him -in its animal, vegetable and mineral forms- and he learned to create a philosophical conscience to try to answer the question that since its very origins have anguished Homo sapiens: Where do we come from, where are we going?

At the same time, as he progressed in his knowledge, that man, from the dawn of time, being initially nomadic and constantly moving throughout his life, came into contact with other men. Whether peacefully or aggressively, invading other people's territories or being subdued by strangers, by hook or by crook, the fact is that there was a gradual exchange of knowledge and practices of all kinds, which enriched the cultural heritage of the different societies.

As in other orders of life, also in the relative one to the health or to its absence, the disease, along with the methods acquired through the practice, tending to conserve the first one, or to remedy the second one, played at the same time a role of great protagonism others of mental nature, fundamentally the magic and the religious ones. It could be said that these filled the void of scientific knowledge, and indeed this is an opinion that has circulated for centuries. But to say such a thing is to oversimplify the issue at hand. It is true that there is a component of empirical ignorance in the use of magic and religion when seeking a cure for the various physical ailments to which man may be subjected and that this use has been manifest since the earliest origins of the human species. Still, it is no less true that such use has generally predisposed the patient to heal. Even today, one still hears everywhere expressions to the effect that the patient himself is his own best physician.

In fact, the patient's state of mind cannot be disregarded in curative practices, even in the most sophisticated hospital of our days. This may be influenced by his humanistic training, his ability to control his mind, religious sentiments, or the most disparate causes. In all cases, whether positively or negatively

Positively or negatively, this will exert a powerful influence on his conscience, achieving, in the first of these cases, a sedative effect, if not effectively curative. It has always been said that faith moves mountains, and this is an enormous component of truth. The fact of wanting to be cured does not cure in itself, perhaps, but it helps greatly when it comes to achieving real healing.

Much of this was already intuited by our ancestors when, along with empirical healing methods, they began to put into practice others of a very different nature. Along with the poultice, the concoction, the massage or the splinting of a fractured bone, the ensalmo, the power of the imagination or the simplest of prayers were applied. It would be difficult today to try to resolve whether it was first cured with empirical methods. On the contrary, it was magic that first played the main role in the most primitive of medicines and then gave way, with time, to scientific practices. It is more likely that the first of these two possibilities occurred: that first, the practical and immediate remedy was sought and then, in the face of its ineffectiveness, the gods or the forces of the unknown, earthly or ultraterrestrial, were invoked to solve this type of problem. Thus, even if it had been discovered that this or that pain could be quickly treated with this or that herb, the other remedies, magical and

3

religious, were not disregarded; who knows if as a reinforcement of the first ones. And, having coexisted together, the latter would have been clearly manifested as having a relaxing and sedative effect with time. It seems that a toothache does less harm if you try to distract yourself by thinking about something else, even if you have taken the appropriate medical remedy.

In summary, let us say that folk medicine is known as the set of empirical and animistic practices aimed at preventing or remedying disease and that in its origins, it was the only medicine known to man. Much later, in a relatively recent period of history and daughter of scientism, a differentiating barrier would be born between medicine understood in the traditional way and imposed through technological advances. However, the basis of the latter would continue to be based in its empirical sense on the content of the former. These days, there has been an attempt to make the gulf between one and the other medicine unbridgeable, generally responding to obscure interests and cataloguing one as rational and praising it, and the other as the daughter of superstition and ignorance and condemning it. Both things are far from reality after analyzing them objectively.

Popular medicine and official medicine

The barrier, which we say is artificial, between popular medicine and scientific medicine, was marked by the medical class itself when it arrogated to itself the privilege of being in possession of the domain of truth. From there to becoming official medicine, there was only one step, always speaking from a historical point of view. And not only did it become the official medicine of the various powers that have divided up the world, but the other medicine became clandestine and outlawed. However, despite its achievements and virtues, the differentiation has not ceased to be unfair, with all due respect to the medicine that physicians apply.

We find ourselves with an unquestioned medical class, with the right to be wrong, owner of bodies and lives, judge of health, self-erected in a powerful monopoly and almost divinized. On the other hand, there are other medicines, the so-called parallel ones, which are rooted in the field of what is known as popular medicine, and which, being different in their substance but above all in their form, are generally much more humanized, are outside the law and have had to survive subject to persecution and slander. Nor should these lines lead us to think that these alternative medicines are the panacea of all wonders, of the most constant successes or the most astonishing miracles. There are successes and failures in both fields, as well as fakers and profiteers who take advantage of the pain of others.

It happens that, in our days, official medicine has provoked weariness and even disenchantment, and several voices have been heard to question it, voices often coming from their own ranks. The phenomenon has coincided with the rise of these parallel medicines, to which many patients have been turning their eyes, to whom orthodox methods gave little hope, especially in the case of ailments considered hopeless.

Of course, distinctions must also be made in this other field. Because at this point, the science that tries to solve health problems by means of methods that are not considered official cannot be called popular medicine either. In general, we are dealing with a type of medicine in which aggressive methods to combat illnesses, such as the use of surgery or the abuse of drugs, rarely appear or are used. This does not mean that such medicines are not scientific, nor that those who practice them do not have academic degrees that accredit their ability. This is the case of the naturalist or naturopathic doctors, of proven solvency in our days and towards whom the eyes are turning at an accelerated pace with fewer doubts. There are also cases of herbalists of recognized international prestige. The same happens with many masseurs, chiro massage therapists, physiotherapists, acupuncturists, and a long etcetera of "different" medical specialities. But, in this case, the origin of their science, wrongly considered modern, comes from popular medicine.

From this popular medicine also comes the presence of chiromancers, ensalmadores, miracle healers and other pseudo-medical variants, who try to treat the disease more through animistic procedures than through the use of empirical methods of a scientific or well-proven nature. In this section are often wrongly placed the current healers, undoubtedly undervalued by urban cultures, which often mistakenly underestimate the scope of their authentic knowledge. There is no doubt that among the so-called healers, there are those of all categories and qualities. Still, it is no less true that, to a large extent, they have tended to become holders of an official medical degree over the course of many decades. However, later, in the practice of their medical functions, they have used atavistic knowledge, or their own experience, when it comes to solving their patients' ailments.

The success of such parallel or unofficial medicines, whether natural, quackery or with religious or magical backgrounds, usually lies in the human warmth. The patient in these cases is not a simple number with a disease of which he understands nothing and of which even the name is often unable to spell. From being a laboratory object or human guinea pig, he usually becomes the main protagonist in the process of his cure, if this is possible, or to find the necessary relief from a condition considered incurable. Because those other medicines, as we say, modern chapter of the popular medicine, besides curing, have tried to humanize the environment of the patient, trying to improve, above all, the quality of life within the evolutionary process of the different ailments, even in irreversible cases or terminal patients.

Some of this was intuited by the village doctors, a figure frequently presented in the literature, with better or worse fortune, but almost never well understood. They were those rural family doctors, an intermediate point between medicine understood in the official way and popular medicine, the latter loaded with superstitions, strange rites and beliefs, which due to their exoticism, have often been considered grotesque. The general practitioner played the role of moderator between practices that were no less harmless in the

6

physical sense but very effective from the point of view of autosuggestion and the spirit, and the scientific methods tested by medical science and known to him. We must not forget that official medicine, as well as the so-called parallel ones, has obtained a good part of its successes by observing popular practices, especially as far as pharmacopoeia is concerned. Almost all the medicines that we know, without the labels that accredit their passage through a laboratory that has experimented with them, have been used in their raw form by all traditional cultures. Even today, they are still used, in the same way, and with similar effects, by numerous primitive peoples.

Healers and other variants of the same profession

The healer has been the one who, many centuries before the official or scientific medicine was imposed, before the family doctor reached every corner of the rural geography, took care, to the extent of his knowledge and his possibilities, to seek healing or relief to the ailments of his neighbours. He did so with greater or lesser success. Still, his figure was so deeply rooted in popular society that he continued to have great prestige even when family doctors and specialists had been completely imposed. So much so that this profession, so subject to contradictory judgments and mistreatment, has not only survived to the present day but enjoys great popularity in very diverse social strata. The reason seems to lie in the great mistrust that, despite advances, medical science continues to inspire in broad social strata, not even among individuals of the highest cultural level.

Today, however, traditional healers, those who acted mainly on faith, the self-taught and those who had inherited their knowledge and their "gift" from their ancestors are becoming scarce. They begin to increase, within the various fields of curanderismo, as we say, healers who practice with the corresponding official medical degree. But this does not mean that anyone could be a healer in the past. On the contrary, it was necessary to meet certain requirements, which fall squarely in the field of superstition and the purest folklore. It was a common belief among most European peoples that a true healer was born with a cross drawn under the tongue or on the roof of the mouth. In addition, it had to be the seventh son, without any female in between. The same happened if the seventh was a daughter and there were no male siblings (although in this regard, this writer has also encountered the opposite belief: that the seventh of the offspring whose siblings were all of the opposite sex was born a curandero, or curandera, the seventh of the offspring). What has not seemed to admit of doubt is that, because of prejudices of different kinds, people have tended to prefer male greeters, except in the case of the midwives. Among very long etcetera of peculiarities, it was also said that the greeters had cried, at least once, when they were still in their mother's womb.

There were different types of healers, depending on their specialities. Although almost all of them were concerned with healing others, some were experts in setting bones and treating rheumatic ailments. Others were skilled in the preparation of potions and ointments. Others knew the secrets of plants inside out. Many of them used exclusively animistic procedures in their cures, such as prayers, ensalmos and religious rituals that, despite being almost always Christian, had a markedly pagan root. Curiously, those that apparently reached the greatest popularity dealt with curing rabies. They proliferated in the villages and were even hired by the town councils. Very characteristic of them was the healing method put into practice on their patients, especially animals, since it was said that they could hold nothing less than boiling oil in their mouths and then throw it with force on the affected person. This therapy gave much to talk about, especially when there were real cases of rabies.

Many have been those who, in one way or another, have lashed out against healers and healers, denouncing the excessive credulity to which they have been subjected. Criticism has proliferated especially from the official medical body, individuals and collectives. For our part, we will neither put nor take away the king, and we leave it to each one to judge for himself.

THE HEAD AND NECK

We already know that a sore head makes thoughts, ideas and intentions run away like a chicken whose throat has been cut. So, to keep always in place, on the shoulders, the more or less fat head that each one has to carry, follow these tips, and you will find that, when the head rules well, the whole body gladly follows.

Against headache

Cut a potato into slices and apply them to the forehead and temples of the patient. Hold with a handkerchief tied to the head.

***

Put cloths of cold water, alcohol or vinegar on the patient's forehead.

***

Pull out four hairs from the patient and place a piece of lead over their roots. Keep the patient fastened with a handkerchief tied to the head.

***

It is also highly recommended to drink the juice of a lemon mixed with the coffee that fits in a cup, naturally without sugar. It is ideal for women's headaches... and men.

***

It may be easier to drink water mixed with pennyroyal, oregano, chamomile and lemongrass (Cymbopogon citratus). This remedy is very fast-acting, as long as the headache is not excessive.

***

Pour vinegar into a cup, dip a white cloth in the vinegar and put it on the patient's forehead until the cloth is dry. At the same time, take an infusion of chamomile very slowly, not too hot. If headaches occur very often, do this operation every day and on an empty stomach. In a week, you will notice the improvement.

**

If the pain is very strong, and although it is somewhat more laborious, put on the fire, in a pan, a clove of garlic in oil and cut it in half. Take out the clove of garlic when it has cooled a little after removing the pan from the fire. Beat an egg white separately and add a handful of chopped verbenas. With the oil lukewarm, pour the egg white with the verbenas into the pan and make an omelette, more juicy than burnt. Wrap the omelette in a cloth and apply it to the patient's forehead until the pain passes.

**

Although much more laborious still, the method considered infallible against stubborn headache is the following: hunt a weasel, burn it once dead, put its hot ashes in a poultice, and put it on the patient's forehead.

Against meningitis

Boil six newborn puppies in a large cauldron, let the patient drink the broth for several days, and he will be cured.

**

Less effective is to place a freshly slaughtered chicken on the neck of the patient, although some assure that it also gives good results.

**

In case of an acute attack of meningitis, a very dangerous ailment, and the patient cannot go to a hospital, place ice cubes on his head, put small pieces of ice in his mouth, and rub his legs vigorously with mustard powder. In the past, this first remedy was reinforced by applying leeches behind the ears.

Against cerebral congestion

Lay the patient with his head high, resting on a horsehair or oat pillow, in neither a cold nor hot room, and apply ice cubes or rags soaked in ice water to his head. In addition, keep him on a diet. To avoid the possible paralysis associated with this condition, act extremely quickly.

***

For those who have already suffered cerebral congestion and are in the process of recovery, administer castor oil - between 30 and 60 grams-or sodium sulfate or magnesium sulfate - between 25 and 40 grams-.

***

Treatment for the recovery of a person who had suffered cerebral congestion was to give him rubs on his legs with mustard powder and apply leeches behind his ears and in his anus.

Against sinusitis

Ingest the affected person, on an empty stomach, the juice of two lemons, mixed with a spoonful of honey.

***

Practice inhalations of eucalyptus while boiling in water for twenty minutes, breathing in through the mouth and breathing out through the nose.

***

Fry a handful of verbena stalks, making sure they are tender, and with them, make an omelette with three beaten egg whites. Place the resulting poultice on a thick white cloth and then on a thinner one, such as gauze. Then apply it all to the affected part of the patient, usually his forehead, and let it cool. Repeat the operation once a day for three consecutive days.

Against sores and inflammation of the gums

Take nine or ten live cockroaches and fry them in a pan with oil. Then strain the oil and touch it to the sore or inflamed gum of the patient. Repeat the operation until the problem disappears.

***

Strain the elderflower, and with the resulting water, gargle and rinse three times a day. To make this remedy more effective, wash the swollen part of the face with the same water.

***

To end a phlegmon, toast flour in a frying pan, put some coals on a plate and over the coals pour a bunch of elder flowers and leaves, blessed on the morning of St. John's Day. Put on a cloth for a couple of minutes so that the vapours moisten it. Soak with the toasted flour the part of the face where the phlegm is, and then put the cloth there. Hold the poultice with a handkerchief knotted to the patient's head. Repeat this until the phlegmon disappears.

***

You can also get rid of phlegmons by smearing them with menstrual blood from a ferret.

***

When the phlegmon hurts, bring the affected person's swollen cheek close to the lock of a door and, through the hole of the door, from the other side, give three blows on the cheek a sietemesinum.

***

It is also of very good effect against phlegmons and mouth inflammations; the following remedy: burn in a pot of dried elderflower, sit the patient on a stool with the pot between the feet, cover with a blanket or sheet the head and receive the steam of the flower for fifteen minutes. Do this as many times as necessary until the phlegm disappears.

Against toothache

Chew incense.

Breathe in vapours of water or boiling milk.

**

Gargle and rinse with an infusion of geraniums.

**

Boil water with three almond shells and three pieces of glass. Gargle and rinse with the water, from which the crystals and almond shells should be carefully removed.

**

Gargle and rinse with boiled acorn water. Do not drink the water.

**

Chew two or three acorns, then let the mass rest on the diseased tooth.

**

Take some tea, some oregano and a glass of wine. Boil well and gargle and rinse.

**

Chew parsley. It is one of the most effective and traditional remedies for toothache.

**

If the teeth hurt, immerse the affected person's feet in hot water to which ash and pepper have been added. If you also add bran, you get an even better effect.

**

Whoever suffers from a toothache, jump on the night of St. John over the typical bonfires, ensuring that the smoke enters his mouth. This will alleviate your ailment throughout the year.

***

If you have problems with your teeth, pick directly from the tree; when it is time, three cherries with your teeth.

Chew in abundance, milongas chestnuts.

***

Place an axe on the side of the face where the toothache is located to relieve the discomfort it causes.

***

If you have a toothache, rinse the affected person with black ox urine.

***

If all else fails, place the affected person on the soles of the feet, two laurel leaves forming a cross. This is an Asturian remedy.

***

To facilitate infant teething, spread oil on the gums of the child.

***

According to popular belief, to keep teeth healthy and clean, nothing is more advisable than biting raw tomato.

Against cold sores and other pupae of the lips.

Rub with an old key while the patient is fasting.

***

Apply a garlic cut in half on the pupa of the lip.

***

Lard-used oil, human urine, and earwax also seem to work well.

***

Collect the affected water from seven different sources for lip fever and store it in a barrel. From each source, collect only one spoonful, and the spoon's owner should be named Maria. Apply this water directly to the affection.

***

To cure cracks in the lips, smear them with a very hot kid tallow.

Against eye irritation

To relieve conjunctivitis, boil several roses, adding a little less than half a teaspoon of sugar to the water. With the resulting liquid, wipe the eyes with a cotton swab. It is also ideal for cleaning the eyes.

***

According to tradition, it is best to take the blessed roses on the day of St. John the Baptist and boil them. When the water is already warm, wet absorbent cotton and wipe the sick eye with it, do this operation as soon as you get up in the morning.

***

Apply a crust of burnt bread, smeared with honey and vinegar, on the sick eye. It is a Galician remedy.

***

Another traditional remedy to cure conjunctivitis is to wash the patient's eyes with the urine of a newborn child. There is a belief in Galician-Portuguese areas, and even in others, that a baby's urine is good for all kinds of ailments or diseases.

***

Wild roses clean the sick eye and protect it from new infections. Therefore, put yourselves in the serene with water and wash your eyes with it in the morning.

***

Boil bramble leaves, which should be left to cool overnight. In the morning, soak a piece of absorbent cotton in it and wipe your eyes with it.

***

Soak a cotton ball in goat's milk and gently rub your eyes with it.

***

Much better still, dip the absorbent cotton in the milk of a woman who is nursing a child, and the eyes and sight will be healed as if by magic.

***

Wipe the eyes with cooked chamomile; it is a very useful remedy against conjunctivitis when you do not have some of the other products at hand, something very frequent, for example, in the city.

***

They say in Alava that if you have bad eyes, the best way to cure them is to touch them with your elbows and not with your hands.

***

If you want to remove any dirt or speck that has entered the inner part of the eyelid, use fine bird feathers. Then wash the eye with warm water.

Against cataracts

According to tradition, some Galicians believe they are cured with poultices of weasel ash.

Against stye

A procedure with cold consists of placing on the stye any of these three things: a metal key of the old ones; the ring of a married woman or widow, applying it nine times in a row, or the sap of a vine branch collected in a glass.

***

A procedure with heat, on the other hand, is to apply a freshly laid hen's egg or mother's milk directly projected from the nipple to the eye or to place over the evil the stocking or sock that the patient has taken off when going to bed, which, or which, is to be kept against the stye all night long.

***

Bathe the lesion with an infusion of blackberry leaves.

***

Wash the stye with water in which a gold coin has been immersed for some time.

***

Dispatch on the granite an egg of a turtle.

***

Wet the lesion with the urine of a virgin twin. Although apparently considered very effective, this remedy was not easy to put into practice due to the suspicion that it could fall on the twin in case it did not take effect.

***

Placing a fly on the stye is undoubtedly simpler, a well-known remedy in Murcian lands.

***

Nor is it difficult as a remedy for this condition, pass over it the tail of a black cat or, even better, if rubbed nine times with the same coinciding with the new moon.

Against earache

Wet the hole of the ear with woman's milk. If the nipple is squeezed directly so that the milk floods the hole, it is said that there is no better remedy against any kind of earache. Some Catalans have gone further and have considered that the remedy is more effective if a patient is a man and the milk is offered by a woman who is breastfeeding a girl. And the other way around, if it is a female patient, the nursing woman must be the mother of a boy.

***

If human milk is not available, use warm olive oil.

***

Bitter almond oil is also effective.

***

As well as oval juice (Withania aristata), according to Canary remedy.

***

After putting two drops of each of these substances in the ear, apply dry heat cloths.

***

A Navarre remedy recommends frying a little parsley in a pan with olive oil and then applying this oil to the pinna that has problems.

***

If what you want is to avoid the annoying ringing that sometimes occurs in the ears after a bath, there is nothing better than putting a pebble in them.

***

To prevent deafness, as long as it is not very pronounced, put a red-hot stone and pour it into a container filled with milk. Apply the resulting steam directly to the diseased ear.

Against ear cooling

If ear cooling occurs due to bad air, place a paper cone in the ear and set it on fire, ensuring that the smoke gets into the ear without burning the patient.

Against nose ailments

To combat sinusitis and nasal blockage, clean three handfuls of finely chopped verbenas in water and let them dry. Then, fry the herbs in oil, and add three beaten egg whites. Mix everything together to make an omelette and place it in a white linen poultice, on which should be placed a gauze. Apply as hot as you can stand on the nose and forehead, and tie with a bandage until it cools. Repeating the operation three times a day, both sinusitis and nasal packing will disappear very soon.

***

Another poultice can be made with the same ingredients but adds a clove of chopped garlic. It goes very well, in addition to sinusitis and nasal packing, for rhinitis or inflammation of the nasal mucous membranes.

To cut nosebleeds

Rub the back of the patient's neck with horsetail infusion and plug the nose with the same plant.

***

Apply vinegar plugs in the nostrils.

***

Throw the patient's head back while raising the arm opposite to the bleeding orifice and plugging the other with the free hand. In some places, it is said to be even more effective if the patient, with the arm corresponding to the bleeding orifice, grasps the ear on the opposite side.

***

Of equal effect is to apply an old iron key on the nape of the neck of the patient, as well as to wet it with cold water, but, of course, without warning him first so that it catches him suddenly.

To get rid of dandruff

Eat raw garlic and an onion every day until dandruff disappears. In addition, with this remedy, the hair will be very strengthened.

***

Collect freshly laid droppings of sparrows and pigeons, put them in boiling water with a clove of split garlic, and once lukewarm, wash the head with the resulting liquid. Rinse the head well afterwards and put on clean hair Agua del Carmen.

***

Another similar remedy is to collect sparrow and pigeon droppings and throw them in boiling water with a clove of broken garlic, but add a glass of sweet anise. Then wash the head with it, let it stand for a few minutes on the scalp, and then rinse the hair. Afterwards, apply Agua del Carmen on the hair.

**

Put on a wreath of roses and wear it on your head for a few days. Then let it dry on the chimney of your house.

**

Pick seven roses from the same branch of a rose bush. Cook with ash in milk, without soap. Put it on your head with a cloth.

**

Cover the head of dandruff with a cap made of vine leaves. Fasten with a handkerchief, knotted at its four ends.

To prevent hair loss

Wet the scalp with a decoction of culantro del Pozo and rub it. It is also recommended to prevent the formation of dandruff.

**

Wash and rinse your head with rosemary water. This will also prevent grey hair.

**

Take some water, a piece of beef, a lot of rosemary and tea leaves. Leave the resulting mixture to rot and pass it over your head.

**

Washing the hair with hot boxwood water also prevents baldness.

Against mumps

Apply warm oil to the patient's neck and wrap a cloth around it.

**

Pass twice the hand of a deceased person who has not yet been buried over the throat affected by mumps, and when the coffin is covered, the evil will go with the dead person to the other world. This curative method, no less known for being unusual, belongs to the British tradition.

Against sore throat in general

Use the eucalyptus in any of these three ways: inhaling the steam given off by its leaves when boiling in a container, on which is placed the head of the patient, covered by a simple towel spread; letting the vapours spread around the room; or sucking candies containing the essence of eucalyptus.

***

Gargle with an infusion of bramble leaves.

***

The same effect is achieved by applying the stocking or sock of the patient's left leg to the neck during the whole night. This procedure is also suitable for hoarseness.

Against angina

Especially when the patient is a child, make him take vapours of dried elderflower, placed on some embers, while keeping his head covered with a towel. Then, put the towel or the cloth used around the neck as a scarf, which should be worn until the pain and inflammation disappear.

***

For angina in children and adults, gargle with an infusion of mallow.

***

One of the most common remedies is still ingested lemon juice.

***

Rinse the mouth, or gargle the patient with water mixed with salt and vinegar.

***

Apply to the patient's neck all night long, the stocking or sock of his left leg, stuffed with roasted bran.

***

Apply to the patient's neck a cloth bag filled with hot wheat bran or hot ash.

***

Apply a poultice prepared from cooking in oil a swallow's nest.

***

Drink four cups of nettle water. Then gargle with marshmallow water, honey and vinegar.

***

Eat a crumbled snake skin, which should be mixed with bran. Although it may seem a very strange remedy, it is very effective.

***

The healer sits the sick person in a chair and places himself in front of him. Rub for one or two minutes with oil on the inner side of the forearm, making crosses on it. Then place yourself behind the patient, cross his arms over his chest and hold his hands so that they protrude from his back. In this way, and while the patient remains embracing himself, slightly fraction the hands so that the self-embrace is intensified.

***

Formerly, in Scotland, they were convinced that the best remedy against angina was for the patient to tie around his neck the rope with which a person had been hanged.

Against larynx or trachea spasms

Ingest three cups daily, outside of meals, of powdered goat's beard or salsify (Tragopogon porrifolius).

***

For laryngitis and pharyngitis, gargle with a decoction of the roots of Campanula rapunculus (Campanula rapunculus).

Against aphonia and hoarseness

Ingest three cups daily, outside of meals, of decoction of culantro del Pozo.

***

Or two cups of sisimbrio or jaramago (Sinapis arvensis) decoction.

***

Drink the hot broth in which two onions have been boiled. This avoids unpleasant snoring at night.

***

More pure licorice.

***

Likewise, let the snorer rinse his mouth and throat with salt before going to sleep.

***

To avoid snoring, take a whole head of garlic, remove only the outer peel and boil slowly in a liter of milk until half remains. Drink before going to bed.

***

Hoarseness can also be avoided by placing a sock full of sawdust or very hot bran around the neck.

THE CHEST

From the chest down, everything can go to hell; we could say if we did not observe some remedies and preventions, which are exposed here, to better care for, and even cure, certain ailments that, neglected, can lead man to the grave. There is no better mirror of man than his chest.

Against any respiratory problem

Provoked vapours of eucalyptus decoction in the bedroom of the sick person.

***

Place a pine tree inside the sick person's room, as close as possible to the bed.

***

Make the patient drink the water in a black horse that has watered.

Against cough and cold

To remove the cough that accompanies the cold, and relieve the symptoms of this one until it disappears, take three infusions of marshmallows, in the morning, afternoon and evening, always outside of meals. It is also highly recommended to macerate the marshmallow in milk and then ingest it in the same amount.

***

Equally effective is the leaf of the cardencha, taken as an infusion three times a day while it is still warm. However, here it is not recommended to macerate the leaves in milk.

***

But since we are talking about milk, boil a good amount of borage in it and drink the resulting decoction three times a day. This remedy also helps to greatly expand the respiratory capacity of any person, healthy or sick.

***

If the cough is very tight to the chest, prepare infusions of cascarilla - the bark of the quinoa tree - to be taken in the same quantity as the previous ones, but in this case, the use of milk is not recommended either. It is a South American remedy.

***

Also, in case the cough is very tight to the chest, that is to say, it is dry, and without sputum, it is more than recommendable the hot wine with honey and the sweetened barley water.

***

More decoctions in red wine: with oregano, marshmallow, barley, walnut leaves and tusilago(Tussilago farfara), known in some areas of northern Spain as horse's claw.

***

It gives very good results also, to make vapours with the decoctions of oregano in milk or vapours of eucalyptus cooked in water.

***

In all cases, it will be very useful to put hot linseed plasters on the chest.

***

Put bags of hot bran on the chest of the person with a cold.

***

Drinking warm donkey's milk helps to expel phlegm.

***

Mix a spoonful of honey and a squeezed lemon for colds in a glass of water. Boil it and drink it as hot as possible. Then, get into bed and wrap up well.

**

Place a small fire in the room of the person who has congestion due to a cold, boil it in water overnight and drink it.

Thyme, rosemary, laurel and eucalyptus in water overnight. There must be a lot of heat and humidity in the room, even if the wallpaper peels off the walls if there is.

**

Against coughs and colds, also take the so-called "snail syrup", whose preparation is as follows: get two dozen snails and six eucalyptus leaves, and put them in a container containing the same amount of water and sugar. Cook and filter through a cloth. The syrup, which will be ready for use, will be kept in a bottle.

**

Another method is to put some alcohol in a dish and set it on fire. While it is burning, throw a cotton compress on it. Immediately cover the plate with another one so that the fire goes out. Take the compress, still warm, and rub the patient's neck or chest with it, as appropriate.

**

It has been believed that it is very good to burn in the house of someone who is constipated, dry bay leaves in a pan.

**

It has also gone very well against coughs, according to popular tradition, to drink milk in which borage flower has been boiled. But for the remedy to have the desired effect, the borage must be cultivated with a golden hoe, and its flower must be collected and dried in the shade.

Against bronchitis

Take garlic decoctions in wine, butter and sugar.

***

Or infusions of ground ivy.

***

If bronchitis becomes acute, take horseradish or strawberry herbal teas.

***

Drink decoctions of thyme with honey and lemon before going to bed.

***

To prevent catarrh and, with it, bronchitis, take daily, on an empty stomach, the juice of a lemon without adding water or sugar. Then eat garlic and onions in large quantities, accompanying meals. Chew parsley to combat bad breath afterwards, which prevents tooth decay.

Against flu and strong constipation

Ingest borage flowers in infusion. Do not despise the combination of milk, honey and cognac, with or without the common aspirin.

***

If the flu is very strong, take three times a day, before each meal, the juice of three lemons without water or sugar.

***

Warm red wine with honey and cinnamon helps to lift the mood and exhaustion caused by the flu. Take after lunch and dinner as a very pleasant dessert.

***

While the flu lasts, eat plenty of lettuce, tomato and carrot salads, to which orange segments and two chopped lemons should be added. Avoid salt, vinegar and oil, which will be replaced by honey.

***

The recommended remedies for coughs and colds are also valid.

To combat pneumonia

To avoid it, cover your neck and chest so that you are safe from the cold of the night.

***

Once pneumonia has taken hold of someone, drink the boiled water of couch grass at least three times a day. It helps to circulate the blood and avoids pulmonary congestion.

***

Whip the patient's back with a bunch of nettles several times a day and for a period of about five minutes each time. Or rub the patient's legs and back vigorously, also with nettles.

***

When the fever that accompanies pneumonia is very high, put on the chest of the patient a poultice made with garlic and cabbage seed.

***

It gives very good results to take decoctions of the tubercles of the tortero, always three times a day.

***

The wolf mint (Lycopus aeropaeus) in poultice, applied on the chest, is equally effective in pneumonia as in pleurisy.

***

As for rubs, those made by rubbing the patient's back strongly with a thick woollen sock or any other woollen garment after having soaked them with alcohol are good against pneumonia.

***

The same must be done with the arms and legs to activate the circulation and avoid pulmonary congestion.

***

Place on the sick person's chest, the offspring of a small animal cut open for twelve hours. If there is no improvement, repeat the operation with another animal. The most convenient pups are those of a dog, cat or rabbit, about six months old. The method can also be used in the case of pulmonary tuberculosis.

***

All the remedies recommended for influenza and catarrh are also valid, which should be combined with the above.

To combat pneumonia

If the sufferer is a man, ingest the urine of a girl of seven years; but if the sick person is a woman, let her drink the urine of a child of the same age.

Against whooping cough

To avoid the convulsions of whooping cough, take fennel infusions at least three times a day. The same with marshmallows. These remedies are especially recommended for children without forgetting the infusion of strawberry leaves, which is even more specific for them.

***

Put on a dowel snail covered with a light coating of sugar. Underneath the dowel, place a vessel that collects the juice distilled, juice to be given to the sick person to drink, by spoonfuls, three times a day.

***

Peel several heads of radish and put them in the serene with sugar. Give the patient the resulting juice to drink.

***

Place a raw onion on the bedside table or under the patient's pillow.

***

Have the patient eat a roasted mouse.

***

If the disease becomes complicated, a traditional remedy has been to move the patient to another place, far away from where he/she was.

***

Another traditional remedy, now discarded, was as follows: the patient was given a sugar cube with a drop of jet fuel on the first day of treatment. Another lump with two drops on the second day, and so on until on the fifteenth day, there were fifteen drops with which the lump was soaked. Thus the treatment was concluded.

Against asthma

The best results have been obtained with asthma patients by placing on the chest, at least three times a day, as all remedies should be administered, cabbage leaves heated over the kitchen fire without burning.

***

The water of cooked ivy leaves is very good and should be mixed with a little elderberry juice. In this case, two tablespoons a day is enough.

***

Also, infusions of orange blossom flowers, thyme, or rosemary, taken at will, are always warm.

**

Put a hot verbena poultice on the sick person's chest until the asthma attack ceases.

**

Likewise, on the patient's chest, apply mustard poultices.

**

Place two cloths on the patient's chest, which must be read, and apply a horse chestnut poultice between them.

**

Pour a small glass of brandy, a little sugar, and a mint and borage thumb into a saucepan. Put it to heat and then drink the resulting decoction. Besides being an excellent remedy against asthma, it is also good against diarrhoea.

**

Loosen the neck, chest and wrists of the patient with a gentle massage. Then rub these parts with a piece of cloth. Rub strongly, first with cold water and immediately with hot water. Then have the sick person get into bed and give him a cup of boiled mallow water to drink. The next morning he will be quite recovered.

**

If the asthma attack is particularly intense, boil a regular-sized onion in a quart of milk until half of the liquid evaporates. Then drink the rest and even eat the onion. The improvement does not take more than ten minutes to come.

**

Whenever possible, take sea baths and breathe the air of the mountains very slowly.

**

A Canarian remedy against asthma consisted of roasting bones of owls, crushing them, boiling them and drinking the resulting broth.

**

It is also a Canarian remedy to boil a puppy a few days old and drink the resulting broth. It is said that a few years ago, a child was cured in this way.

**

Others, however, prefer to drink for at least three days the broth where a black cat has been boiled.

**

They also say that those who eat carrots in abundance never suffer from asthma.

Against tuberculosis

There is nothing better against tuberculosis, even when the disease has been declared in its most advanced stage, than to ingest raw dandelion herb at the discretion and preferably in large quantities. Above all, the dandelion herb or bitterroot resembles a starfish (Taraxacum officinale).

**

The juice of jaramagos, a remedy against widespread disease in tropical areas, is also recommended, although only in the amount of one glass per day.

**

Do not take animal fats or meat; only fruits, cereals and vegetables.

**

Make abundant ingestion of raw lemon juice.

***

Eat plenty of seasoned but tender beans with olive oil.

***

Make a decoction of sage, celandine and verbena, sweeten with honey and take it on an empty stomach.

***

Take infusions of sorrel (Rumex Crispus).

***

Ingest the green bark of the walnut fruit, macerated with consecrated wine.

***

Macerate two chicken eggs with their shells in plenty of lemon juice, and drink it all afterwards.

***

Ingest on an empty stomach the urine recently expelled by a one-year-old child, a remedy well known since ancient times by all Indo-European peoples.

***

Remedy already in disuse against tuberculosis consisted of preparing the following poultice: fry verbena leaves and passes them through a silk cloth or similar. Place the cloth, with the leaves inside, on the patient's chest and add an egg yolk on top. Cover the whole thing with a gauze or bandage. Do this before going to bed and keep it on all night. Repeat the operation several nights in a row, and it will be observed that one morning the cloth will appear stained with blood and pus. Continue the treatment until all the evil is gone.

THE CIRCULATION

The body is like a car and even a train, powerful and beautiful if it is cured when it is necessary to do so and if those circulatory blockages are prevented that do not allow the blood to run through the veins with all its oxygen and with all its nourishment of the body. As we know: let the blood flow. And think that you have for your heart a bonbon.

For blood pressure

In order to keep your blood pressure normal and neither rise nor fall, take frequent infusions of the roots and leaves of aladierna (Rhamnus alaternus), which help the blood circulation to be more fluid.

***

Also, take infusions of branches, trunks and roots of sloe berries, which help to level high blood pressure.

***

Boil wild olive branches, let the resulting product macerate and take a teaspoon of it every morning.

***

It also gives very good results in the infusion of carrasquilla or guillomo (Amelanchier Canadensis), as well as the infusion of Centaurea minor (Centaurium erythraea).

***

It is no longer recommended to bleed the arms of patients with hypertension, as in the past.

***

An excellent hypotensive, and that is also a wonderful tonic for the heart; we have it in the nettles, which ingested in decoction give very good results to level blood pressure.

***

The infusion of hawthorn, also called hawthorn (Crataegus monogyna), also corrects high or low blood pressure. In general, it is excellent as a cardiac tonic.

***

Mistletoe herbal teas are especially recommended.

***

And although it may seem strange, ingest for three days, every morning and on an empty stomach, a glass of water with chimney soot only if you suffer from high blood pressure.

***

An excellent method to regulate blood circulation and level blood pressure is to take three infusions of celandine or swallowwort (Chelidonium majus) a day.

***

For the same, put five walnut leaves in a quart of water, and then cook everything until only half of it is left. Drink on an empty stomach.

Also, take infusions of couch grass root.

***

Bathe your feet and hands in an infusion of mallow, rosemary and greater plantain.

***

Put your hands and wrists in cold water to lower your blood pressure when it is high.

***

Against low blood pressure, an excellent method is also to eat spinach or chicory in abundance.

***

A remedy already in disuse was to take infusions of lesser celandine. But it had to be done with caution since this plant contains toxic substances.

This plant contains toxic substances.

***

Eat raw pork spleen, even if it is disgusting. It favours blood circulation.

***

To maintain normal blood pressure, take sea baths an odd number of times, for example, five, seven, nine, etc...

To alleviate heart ailments

For those who suffer from heart disease, whatever their illness, it is advisable to eat fried hake liver and take rosemary infusions.

***

A good remedy for all heart ailments: boil in the water a few branches of blackthorn (Prunus spinosa). Drink the water resulting from the cooking in a cup, always on an empty stomach, for at least a week.

***

Boil in the water a sliver of blackthorn (Amelanchier Canadensis), and then drink the water in a cup, in the morning and on an empty stomach, for no more than four days.

***

Eat a lot of garlic with meals, or take it raw at any time.

***

Drink an infusion made with orange leaf, orange blossom, rue and wild olive tree three times a day.

***

For nervous palpitations, ingest infusions of rue, lemon balm (Melissa officinalis), jume (Suaeda divaricata), herb Clin (Ajuga iva), and orange and orange blossom leaves.

***

Whoever suffers from heart palpitations will feel relief just by putting a metal key in his mouth.

***

Against tachycardia, take infusions of juniper flowers.

***

Against cardiopathies in general, order the healer to kill two hens. Rip out the heart of one of them, pierce it with pins and bury it. When it rots, the sick person will be healed. Take the other hen with you.

Against anaemia

Put a few wormwood herbs in half a glass of wine, let it macerate overnight, and drink the resulting liquid on an empty stomach in the morning.

***

Drink as much ferruginous water as possible.

***

In the case of anaemic children, give them unboiled donkey's milk to drink.

***

A very good remedy is a preparation based on egg yolk with its pulverized shell, sugar and raw lemon juice. The mixture should be left overnight and taken on an empty stomach the next morning.

***

Make a decoction of oak bark and drink the resulting liquid as often as desired.

***

Or take decoctions of grated bark of caper root.

***

Rub the anaemic person's back with a mixture of eggs and sherry wine.

***

To prevent anaemia, eat abundant and strong food, being parsley always present in the dish.

***

In Castile, they used to say that the best way to avoid anaemia was to drink fresh bull's blood, and even better if the bull was a fighting bull.

Against rickets or softening of the bones

Ingest Cardamine juice, also called prat cress (Cardamine pratensis).

***

Eat stewed dog puppies in abundance.

Against diabetes, cholesterol and uric acid

Collect argoma flowers and let them dry in an airy place, in the shade. Take in infusion when convenient.

***

Drink the liquid resulting from the decoctions of walnut leaves or artichokes. The second of these remedies are ideal for diabetes.

**

Pick argoma flowers, let them dry in the shade in an airy place, and then ingest an infusion made with them.

**

Add 100 grams of parsley to a liter of white wine and, in a bottle, let it stand for twelve days. After this time, drink a glass of this wine before meals. It is also an excellent remedy to lower cholesterol and uric acid.

It fights diabetes by ingesting parsley on an empty stomach.

**

It is also good to end diabetes by taking the juice of the becabunga (Veronica beccabunga).

**

Likewise, against diabetes, the patient should take the gall of a chicken. As it is extremely bitter, help with a sip of water.

**

Take a decoction of walnut leaves and bark, but outside of meals.

**

Drink infusions of centaurea or gall of the earth.

**

In order to know if a person had diabetes, in the Canary Islands in the past, they were made to drink the boiled water of yerba clin without sugar. If he found it sweet, he had diabetes; if he found it bitter, he did not.

**

In general, against cholesterol, the ingestion of parsley in abundance has traditionally been recommended.

***

If you do not want to have excess cholesterol, eat four or five nuts a day.

***

It also helps to control cholesterol, the ingestion of oranges or their natural juice as much as you want.

To combat gout

Take two cups daily of the decoction of alquejenje (Physalis alkekengi) between meals.

***

Or two cups, one in the morning and one in the evening, of cane decoction.

***

Walk the affected person barefoot on the grasses wet by the dew of dawn. It is even better if he does it on the morning of St. John's Day.

***

Take infusions of tomato seeds and leaves, or drink a lot of tomato juice.

***

Ingest decoctions of reinette apples, sugar and honey.

***

Drink infusions of lime blossom and mint.

***

Infusions of ash leaves are also good. It is recommended to take them before going to sleep.

To combat arthritis

If it is chronic, take ash leaves in infusion, mixed with lemon juice and a teaspoon of honey.

***

Ingest decoctions of wild apple bark.

***

Rub the patient in the affected areas with nettle bushes.

***

Introduce the patient, one by one, the arthritic fingers inside a fresh egg, with a hole made in its upper part, and keep them inside until it has warmed up well.

Against phlebitis

Ingest two cups of horse chestnut infusion daily, as this plant has vasoconstrictive properties.

For the blood in general

The carrot in boiling - the so-called carrot water - is one of the best remedies known to keep the blood clean and fresh.

***

Make yourself abundant ingestion of lettuce leaves, which contain precious oxygen to make the blood irrigation more fluid.

***

Take hot and cold showers, alternating one and the other.

***

To combat the impurities of the blood, take infusions in which you have boiled rosemary, thyme and chamomile, divided into equal parts.

***

Also, purify the blood infusions of blackberry and vine leaves, especially if it is red.

Against piles

Drink cold water while applying linseed, marshmallow and poppy plasters on the affected area. Alternatively, soothe the piles with vapours of cardamom water and with warm water enemas.

***

Wet the piles with fasting saliva or with lye.

***

Boil horsetail (Equisetum arvense) and then apply it to the piles. You can also drink the liquid.

***

Make a decoction of the roots of cinquefoil or cinquefoil (Potentilla reptans), drink the liquid and apply part of it to the piles.

***

Apply directly to the piles with absorbent cotton and blackberry decoctions.

***

Do the same with the liquid of walnut and thyme decoctions.

***

Apply bacon and garlic to the sore anus.

***

Rub the same delicate place with oil in which prickly pears have been fried.

***

Apply on the anus during the whole night; a tomato opened in half.

***

Take hot sit vapours. There are many kinds, such as cooking chamomile, wheat bran or smoke from burning leeches.

Drink infusions of brown leaves. Take decoctions of horse chestnuts.

Or onion bulb (Allium schoenoprasum).

***

A very old remedy is to sit, bare-assed, on a frog opened in half.

***

According to a popular oriental belief, eat a lot of dates if you do not want to have piles.

Against varicose veins

Take the shells of twelve snails, but ensure they are still alive. Put them on the soles of the feet and wrap them in a cloth so that the snails remain in contact with the skin. Then cover the foot with a plastic bag. This poultice will be maintained during the whole night, and the same operation should be repeated for several nights in a row until the varicose veins of the extremities disappear, or what is the same, until the snails begin to appear stained with the blood of almost black color.

***

Rub your feet and legs with walnut water.

***

Put on legs and feet the juice of the herb blackberry or Santa Maria (Solanum nigrum), and rub gently over the affected area. Avoid ingestion, as it is highly toxic.

***

Drink decoctions of new elm leaves, but outside of meals.

***

Or horse chestnut decoctions, but no more than a couple of cups a day.

The most necessary depurative

Nothing is better than taking frequent infusions of borage and marshmallow to make the blood purification that the body requires from time to time.

***

Also, ingest daily the juice of one or two raw lemons without water or sugar.

***

Take, even from time to time, infusions of horsetail.

***

Drink infusions of rosemary, thyme or chamomile at your discretion.

***

Take decoctions of verbena leaves and white nettle indistinctly.

Bloodletting and leeches

Avoid such uses, because although very popular in the past, they can offer more dangers than benefits. Moreover, the World Health Organization has expressly forbidden them.

THE BELLY

He whose belly goes well, the better off he will be. Yes, of the belly and the concomitant parts, as a healer from Cordoba (Argentina), a great expert in the value of many herbs, used to say. With the belly, it is the same as with the chest. From the belly and those concomitant parts, we must make health so that life goes on.

Against pain and heartburn

It has been observed that drinking sea water in small quantities and every day preserves the stomach from the evils that are proper to it, facilitates the evacuation and makes the digestion lighter, no matter how copious the meals are made.

***

To combat heartburn, drink a glass of warm milk with an egg beaten in it. Some Basque healers recommend adding to this a glass of pacharan.

***

Another excellent remedy consists of taking a glass three times a day with the decoction of clover roots.

***

For stomach pain, apply a linseed compress on the stomach, which will be made with milk or red wine; if necessary, it should be worn for as long as the pain persists, knotted with a cloth as a girdle.

***

Rub the stomach strongly, making pressure from top to bottom with the thumbs.

***

A remedy of the magical tradition says it is very good to put a coin on the stomach, with the face inward and the cross outward.

**

Put candle wax and tow in a glass. Place the bottom of the glass on the stomach: the wax will attract the pain, and the tow will dilute it.

**

Rub the stomach with brandy and soap that has not yet been used. Let the mixture dry. Wash when the pain has passed.

**

Apply on the stomach, but a little towards the right side of the body, plasters of bacon herb, or rue, or rosemary, solidified with olive oil, butter and wine.

**

Equally useful are plasters made of linseed meal kneaded with milk.

**

In general, verbena cloves, eaten in salads, raw lemon to heal ulcers, and warm verbena herbal teas are very useful.

**

Do not disregard, whenever the stomach hurts, an infusion of clover, fennel, or ground ivy, because they relieve immediately and facilitate the digestion of what is eaten later.

Against gastritis

Take infusions of flowers and leaves of common mallow.

**

When it is mild, sugar calms it. In case of persistence or increasing intensity, crumble rhubarb roots and put them in a bottle with water, which should be kept closed for a few days. The dose will be that of glass, drunk three times.

***

A mother and a daughter collect three handfuls of earth from three graves in the same cemetery and mix them with diluted homemade chocolate. Then give it to the patient to eat.

Against stomach or duodenal ulcers

Take infusions of yarrow (Achillea millefolius), but without the plant's root.

***

Ingest decoctions of mallow and barley in equal parts.

***

Do the same with common chamomile and chamomile called Roman or noble chamomile (Chamaemelum nobile).

***

Infusions of nettles are not bad either. The ideal is to drink the first one on an empty stomach, another one at mid-afternoon and the last one a while before going to bed.

***

Excellent is also the decoctions of alchemilla leaves or lion's foot (Alchemilla Vulgaris).

Against stomach decay

Heat in a dish with a little brandy. Separately, crumble on a linen cloth and it some Maria cookies. Melt the hot brandy on both products and fold the cloth so that everything is inside. Apply in this way on the pit of the stomach.

***

Apply a linen compress soaked in brandy to the pit of the stomach.

For any disorder of the belly

Eat thyme soup. It is a tradition that this plant has special virtues if it is collected on Holy Thursday and Good Friday and, even more, if the time of collection is midnight, which goes from one day to the other mentioned.

***

Against the hardening of the belly, boil watercress in water. Remove the water and fry it in butter when the watercress cools down. Place on the patient's belly wrapped in a cloth.

***

Call a twin to rub the patient's belly, stomach and kidney area for a gastrointestinal problem with fried olive oil. Then beat him with a cloth soaked in cold water. Repeat the operation for three consecutive days

***

If the belly hurts, take a pigeon and cut it open. Without even plucking it, apply it to the patient's belly, and hold it until it begins to smell rotten, at which time the treatment is finished.

***

If a breast-fed child suffers from intestinal colic, when breast-feeding him, place his mother across him so that the child's body, legs outward, forms a cross with hers.

For spleen problems

If the sufferer is a child, take the patient to a meadow where there is a walnut or mulberry tree, and place him under either of these trees, standing and stepping on herbs of lesser plantain. Cut away with a knife the earth around the child's feet, and place the clod at the level of the patient's spleen, on the outside of the shirt. Then have the child return home and force him/her to enter through a door other than the one he/she left, or through a window, if the house has only one door. When the clod dries, the child will be healed.

***

Apply a poultice of cow dung to the side while it is still warm.

***

To avoid engorgement of the spleen and the characteristic pain that some know as "limaco", place three stones on the floor, one on top of the other, and give the affected person three laps with his hands around them.

***

Or stop who feels pain in the spleen, bend down and pick up a stone from the ground, then stand up again, wet it with saliva or kiss it and place it on the ground again. The pain will disappear as if by magic.

To whet your appetite

Take one or two cups a day of white acacia bark decoction.

***

Drink three cups of chicory root decoction a day, but outside of meals.

***

Drink a cup of infusion of savoury when getting up, on an empty stomach, and another one a while before going to bed.

***

Against infantile malnutrition, in some areas of Castile, the child has been given to eat bread soups cooked in owl broth, although the meat of the slaughtered animal was not eaten.

***

However, others are of the opinion that the lost appetite is also recovered by eating owlets in abundance.

Against bad breath

Take infusions of sorrel leaves.

*****

Drink infusions of caraway fruits also called meadow cumin (Carum carvi).

*****

Drink infusions of the root of archangelic, also known as Carlina (Archangelica officinalis).

*****

Or common mint.

To avoid vomiting

In general, and when nausea and vomiting are continuous, take chamomile water with half a glass of brandy, anise or pacharan. In the British Isles, they add half a glass of whiskey to a cold tea.

*****

They always give very good results the mint decoctions or tea with mint in the North African Arabian style.

*****

When nausea is persistent, and there is no emission of vomit, an infusion of feverfew (Tanacetum parthenium) immediately prevents spasms.

*****

Equally recommended is the tisane of greater celandine.

*****

If nausea does not subside and the patient feels that he/she should vomit but does not vomit, drink warm milk with vinegar.

***

Take linseed soap, water or marshmallows to cut vomiting and stop nausea.

To induce vomiting

Insert the index and middle fingers under the uvula and on the tongue of whoever needs it.

***

Take vinegar and, once vomiting has occurred, milk.

***

Especially in cases of drunkenness, drink very salty coffee.

***

If the drunkard is on the verge of an ethyl coma, make him smell ammonia.

To avoid dizziness

If a woman is prone to travel sickness, place a bunch of parsley in the hollow between her breasts.

***

Cover the navel with a bandage if you do not want to get dizzy.

***

You can also avoid dizziness by placing a sprig of parsley in the anus.

***

If it occurs at sea, chew salted cod at the slightest symptom.

Against fainting

To bring the affected person back to his senses, rub his temples and nose with vinegar.

Against drunkenness

If you have drunk a lot of alcohol, eat some garlic soup afterwards.

***

Although, according to popular tradition, the best thing for a drunkard is to make him drink eagle's blood (today, a protected bird, by the way, as surely no one should ignore).

***

If you want an alcoholic to hate drinking, make him drink bitch's milk.

Against hiccups

Drink sips of water, holding your breath and in an odd number of times.

***

Frighten the hiccups, or make them startle for any reason.

***

Stare at any point, and this discomfort will disappear.

***

Turn the affected person any garment inside out.

***

Sniff tobacco powder to provoke sneezing, which will make the hiccups disappear.

***

If the sufferer is a breastfeeding child, put a pulverized coffee bean in the mouth between the fingers. Then give him/her a little water or milk.

***

Or give the child a large spoonful of water with a drop of aniseed or a spoonful of aniseed water.

Against constipation

If the sufferer is a breastfeeding child, insert a little parsley in the anus.

***

Or rub the anus with the head of a match impregnated with olive oil or with absorbent cotton soaked with this same product.

Apply an enema with grass water.

***

Perform enemas with chamomile water and a splash of olive oil.

***

Ingest starch diluted in water and betony herbal teas (Betonica Officinalis).

***

Take decoctions of holly leaves.

***

Mulled wine drunk in very small sips or taken in spoonfuls gives very good results.

***

Drink a seaweed decoction.

***

If constipation is persistent, use infusions of mallow root with a few grains of salt and a few drops of oil.

*****

Also recommended are Plantago psyllium seeds macerated in aniseed.

*****

The spurge plants (Euphorbia lathyris), consumed in cooking, help evacuate quickly.

*****

Centaurea infusions, known as earth gall (Centaurium erythraea), also help to have a bowel movement without problems.

*****

In the early morning, go out on the balcony without clothes from the waist down and stay there until you feel the effects of the cold in your stomach. The next morning, as soon as you wake up, drink a glass of water that was left in the evening in the serene, covered with a cloth so that it does not get dirty.

*****

Leave a glass of water, covered, during the whole night in the evening and drink it in the morning on an empty stomach.

*****

Or drink water with a little oil.

*****

Try to act as a stabbed body because this way, the pressure of the muscles of the belly on the anus is greater. If you do not have a Turkish bowl, pen, or a place nearby where you can do it, squat on the common toilet bowl.

*****

If nothing better is available, drink sea water in long gulps.

***

If constipation is chronic, drink one or two cups of white acacia bark decoction daily.

***

Or, if it is the season, eat plums in abundance.

Against intestinal obstruction

Practice on the abdomen of the patient a good massage with the thumbs of the thumbs until you find the place of the obstruction, which is at the same time the one of maximum sensitivity. The massages should be centred there, directing them from the pit of the stomach parallel to the edge of the ribs. To perform them, the masseur should use oil with chamomile. But if the pain is very intense at the mentioned point, or the person gets worse, it will be necessary to abandon the massages since it can be a serious injury. If this circumstance does not occur, after the massages are finished, place a coin on the navel of the patient, a lighted candle on it and cover both things with glass. When the flame of the candle is extinguished for having extracted the bad airs, a handkerchief dipped in rum and fastened with a fork should be tied around the patient's waist. Previously, and in a repeated way, it will have been flamed, taking care that it does not burn. This handkerchief will be covered with a cloth or flannel and fastened to the belly with a strong bandage. At the same time, the patient will be given a cup of sweetened chamomile and a glass of rum. An hour later, the patient will eat a good meal, with a predominance of white bread, a roast cutlet and aged wine. Things that, on the contrary, he will have to abstain from the tasting are beans, broad beans, pork products and viscera of any animal.

***

The method of swallowing two round 16 calibre rifle bullets is not recommended at all. Previously, it was proved that the one swallowed in second place tended to come out through its natural duct before the one swallowed in the first place. The disadvantage of this therapy was that if the digestive tract was obstructed as a result of a serious ailment, for example, a cancer of the esophagus, the remedy could be fatal. There were also many disadvantages if, instead of round bullets, elongated bullets were used, as they could be crossed, forming a cross inside the organism.

To avoid bad gases

To avoid aerophagia or farts, drink infusions of the fruits of caraway, also called meadow cumin (Carum carvi).

***

Also, infusions of mugwort of the Alps (Artemisia genipi), taken in two or three cups daily, but outside meals, are not bad.

***

Nor the infusions of asperilla (Galium odoratum), but without abusing them.

***

Against the formation of gases, apply on the stomach poultices of eggs.

***

Or an omelette made with rue, rosemary and sage, very hot.

***

Although used in the past by a healer from Guipuzcoa to remove bad air, the following remedy is not recommended: it consists of massaging the patient in the belly, from bottom to top, while blowing strongly through the anus. For the method to be effective, verifying that the patient expels the air by the mouth is necessary.

***

57

Another Basque remedy against intestinal gas is the following: with the tips of the thumbs, massage intensely on the belly. If this does not achieve the objective, making a hot chocolate poultice will be necessary to force the gases to come out through the navel. To facilitate this operation, place a coin on the navel of the patient, and on it a lighted candle, all of which will be covered with glass. The remedy will be finished the moment the flame of the candle is extinguished. The treatment should be repeated for twelve or fifteen days.

Against indigestion

Take infusions of tarragon leaves and buds (Artemisia dracunculus).

***

If it is a child who suffers from it, place a live fish on the navel.

Against colic and stomach pains

The best thing to do for stomach pains is to apply heat to the area. But if the pain does not subside soon, leave the heat aside and go to a specialist because in the case of appendicitis, the contact of heat not only will not help but will aggravate the condition.

***

If a clear hardening of the belly accompanies the pain in the stomach, boil watercress in water, remove the water afterwards, then fry the watercress in butter and, putting it in a cloth as a poultice, put it on the belly.

***

An Indo-European tradition indicates that whoever suffers from stomach aches should drink his urine every morning. It is said that Gandhi used to do it.

***

As strange as it may seem, a very good remedy is to drink chicken excrement water, but only for men. For women, chamomile and brandy are recommended.

***

Very useful plasters are made with verbena tortillas or chamomile fried with oil, which are put on the affected area.

Against colic, the infusion of fennel is very useful.

***

Also, the moderate ingestion of fennel, cucumber, cherry liqueurs, and apple liqueur.

***

Nuts macerated in aniseed soothe the pain of colic, which are also an excellent dessert, carminative and very suitable for good digestion.

Against diarrhea

Take pure lemon juice as often as necessary until diarrhea stops.

***

Ingest pujo flower or yarrow infusions, or what is the same, Achillea millefolius.

***

Rice water, or rice with milk, lemon and white wine, is an extraordinarily good and quick remedy for diarrhea, as long as neither sugar nor honey is added. The modern saccharin is fine to use.

***

Take starch diluted in water.

***

Beat an egg white in white wine, and then take it at least three times a day until diarrhea disappears.

**

Make a liqueur based on brandy, sugar, mint and borage. Tradition recommends making it in summer and under the sunlight. It is very useful and pleasant to drink after meals, also as a digestive tonic.

**

Make decoctions of cinquefoil or cinquefoil (Potentilla reptans), or sloes or pacharanes, which are very astringent. Drink the liquid resulting from these decoctions.

**

Drink infusions of comfrey root (Symphytum officinale).

**

Drinking water of nisperero, quince, guava or pennyroyal mint buds is highly recommended.

**

Blackberry wine is also a more than effective remedy, which also immediately removes the pain of cramps.

**

Drink a glass of half beer and half water.

**

Drinking beer with sugar and eating quince jam is also very effective.

**

In the past, diarrhea was avoided by drinking white wine in which the white of an egg was mixed. Afterwards, an enema prepared with linseed water, mallows and corn leaves was applied.

**

In the popular world, both against diarrhea and constipation, it is common to use apples, either cooked or raw.

Against colitis

Ingest three cups daily, outside meals, of powdered goat's beard or salsify (Tragopogon porrifolius).

***

Or two teaspoons daily of infusion of onion bulb (Allium schoenoprasum).

***

Take infusions of the strawberry root.

***

Or decoctions of parietaria.

***

In addition to massaging the belly, women should take a decoction of chamomile with brandy, and men should take a decoction of chicken droppings.

To combat worms

There is nothing better for children and adults with parasites than ingesting tisanes of plantain.

***

Very beneficial are also infusions of wormwood, as well as decoctions of walnut leaves and infusions of holly leaf taken on an empty stomach.

***

Tisanes made with male plantain, and laurel decoctions in milk are also excellent. They can be drunk or taken as a sitz vapour with them.

Infusions of feverfew are also recommended.

***

Popular tradition dictates that children with worms should be hung around their necks with a necklace made with garlic.

***

Since ancient times, it has been known that plum and walnut pericarp liqueur fight intestinal parasitism to the thousand wonders.

***

But perhaps it is more effective to drink soot water, or to ingest, always on an empty stomach, a teaspoonful of olive oil.

***

Put nettle plasters on the stomach of the sick person.

***

Even if it is not pleasant, drink half a liter of milk, in which half a dozen peeled garlic has been boiled.

***

Apply on the belly poultices of garlic cooked in milk or fried in oil.

***

Another well-known and effective remedy since ancient times is lying the sick person face down and placing a piece of raw meat over the anus. It will not take long for the parasites to come out, attracted by the smell of fresh meat.

***

It is also recommended to ingest raw or cooked garlic or the water from its decoction.

***

An Asturian remedy consists in applying raw garlic to the patient's neck and celery on the chest and making him drink decoctions of peppermint.

Against tapeworm

Sit the patient in a chamber pot full of milk and wait until the tapeworm makes its exit to the outside through the anus. If this does not occur, repeat the operation as often as conveniently.

***

The remedy will be more effective if, in addition, the patient ingests pumpkin seeds in abundance.

***

Purge the patient at night with three large spoonfuls of castor oil. On an empty stomach, take a handful of ground pumpkin seeds mixed with sugar in the morning. Two hours later, take the same amount of castor oil again as in the evening.

***

If the tapeworm or tapeworm is not expelled, reinforce the remedy with 50 grams of dried pomegranate bark, left to macerate in water overnight, and the patient will drink on an empty stomach the next morning after boiling it for a few minutes and then allowed to cool. The patient should have breakfast two hours later, and his problem will have disappeared.

Against liver ailments

To avoid them, eat few or no eggs and beware of eating pork, especially pork liver, which is very toxic.

***

Because of the whey, it contains milk preserves from contracting liver diseases.

***

Thermal waters and whey give magnificent results in the treatment of liver diseases.

Against hepatitis

Take infusions of chicory and Parietaria at will, as long as the disease lasts.

Against jaundice

A very traditional remedy is to make the patient, without his knowledge, eat a common louse, according to this recipe: put in a jar of chocolate, or mixed in a soft liquor, several lice, seven, nine, eleven, thirteen ... always in the quantity that makes nones. The lice' aim is to break the supposed membrane that does not allow the bile to flow, producing jaundice.

***

A similar remedy consists in drinking a glass of water in which seven head lice have been put.

***

In Galicia, to cure the same disease, they give the patient, for nine consecutive days, a glass of wine with nine lice, which has been previously left to the Sereno. For the remedy to be effective, the patient must drink it on an empty stomach.

***

It was also said that jaundice was cured simply by the patient watching the water run. For this, nothing more recommendable than throwing pebbles from a bridge into the current of a river, and even better if he did it on an empty stomach and on a Friday. In other places, they have thrown chickpeas on the morning of San Juan.

***

Drink corn water, or crumble verbena in the contents of a bottle of white wine. Taking three small glasses a day, jaundice disappears in a short time, and the liver is cured.

***

Drink donkey milk.

Drink also the water from corn husks.

***

Or rosemary infusions.

Against gallstones

If you suffer from gallstones, take ash leaves in infusion, mixed with lemon juice and a teaspoon of honey.

Prolapsus of the rectum

They are a disease that usually occurs in the elderly and in children who are forced to make enormous efforts to make belly because of constipation. Healing tradition dictates that the patient be treated with what is necessary to prevent constipation. If the patient manages to have a bowel movement without straining, the annoying prolapsed bowels will disappear.

To combat dropsy

Against fluid retention was formerly used to tie a pink ribbon around the waist and follow for nine days a diet based on donuts and sweet wine.

***

If the sick person was a child, another tradition ordered, at least in Navarre, to rub the navel with oil brought by five old widows from five different churches.

***

According to a Galician remedy, put the sick person in bed, naked and with a piece of brown paper on the belly, and make crosses on the paper with a knife or with scissors dipped in oil, but gently to avoid causing a wound.

***

A very old custom orders to open a live hen in half and put it on the belly of the sick person.

***

It is also not bad to take cane decoctions, a cupful on an empty stomach in the morning, and another one a while before the patient goes to sleep.

***

Take the patient to a hill from which the sea can be seen and lay him down on the ground. Mark the outline of his body on the ground, collect the corresponding clods and take them home to burn them in the hearth fire. As the clods dry, the sick person will be healed.

***

But in the case of a condition related to circulation and fluid retention, it is best to use the remedies specified here in the section dedicated to the ills of the circulation. Or to those that speak of depurative remedies.

To cure hernias

Here also the magical and religious tradition has commanded. For example, three twigs were planted in the ground. If they took root, the sick person was cured; if they did not, he died.

***

However, the most widespread remedy in the popular world was to bundle the sick person.

Against infantile hernias

Gather three persons named John the Baptist, on the night of the eve of St. John, shortly before the stroke of midnight, near an oak tree. Curve up the tree and, while the twelve bells are ringing, pass the three Johns to the hernious, one to the other, over the tree, while saying: "-Take it, Baptist". "-Give it to me, Baptist". "-Take it, Baptist..." The operation has to be carried out in the absolute secrecy. It is a formula that belongs to the magical tradition, but, in a more natural order of things, and since it is a serious injury, it would be best to take

The best thing to do is to take the child to a medical specialist.

***

On the other hand, the operation in the Canary Islands was carried out by passing the small hernious child through a mimbrero, and a John, an Elizabeth and a Mary had to intervene. The operation is as follows: at dawn on St. John's day, simultaneously open a wicker rod from a bush facing the sea and the mountain. Take the herniated child, Mary, and pass it inside the cut rod for John to pick it up on the other side while he asks: "-What do you give me, Mary?" "-A broken child", -Mary answers- "-St. John and the Virgin give him to be healthy," -John will add-. Say the same words repeatedly while passing the child from one hand to the other, and repeat the operation for another two years. Join the wicker rod again; if it does not dry up, the sick person will be healed.

***

This is a tradition known throughout Europe, with slight variations. In some regions, holm oaks, ash or cork oaks are used; in others, cherry, pear, olive, walnut, poplar or rose trees, among longer etcetera.

***

However, here again, in the case of a hernia, it is necessary to consult a medical specialist for the necessary remedies. It is a serious condition, the neglect of which can have unfortunate consequences for those who suffer from it.

THE URINARY TRACT

He who does not pee does not need to wiggle either, as the saying goes. With this, we only want to point out how important it is to urinate well, long and gladly, to keep the body's plumbing in good condition, those that also provide other pleasures. And for women: She who does not pee well will always be ugly.

To prevent children from wetting the bed

First of all, and according to the oldest popular thought, so that children do not pee in their sleep, they should not play with fire, light bonfires, not even very small ones, or handle lighters, matches, flares or firecrackers.

***

But if, in spite of everything, they urinate in the middle of the night, give them to drink, for nine days in a row, water in which a mole has been boiled.

***

In case the procedure does not work either, give them a decoction of three handfuls of earth from a cemetery, collected from the grave of the last deceased. For the treatment to be effective, the patient mustn't know what he is ingesting, so the product should be conveniently mixed with flour or other foods.

***

The simplest method, however, is sure to make the patient keep his feet submerged in hot water nine nights in a row for the time necessary to recite five Our Fathers and five Hail Marys. Then take five steps in a dry place and get into bed.

***

These remedies belong to the magical and religious tradition, and as faith moves mountains, as you know: let each one put his grain of faith or sand.

***

However, it has been proven that for children who wet the bed without being old enough to do so, it is very good to give them an infusion of lime blossom in the middle of the afternoon. A few days later, the sheets will be dry when it is time to get the child up for school.

To urinate without problems

Peeing many times a day means that the kidneys are working perfectly. So, to get the kidneys going like washing machine pumps, which is what they really are, drink plenty of water, at least two liters a day.

***

Take infusions of Arenaria or stone-breaker (Herniaria glabra) to cleanse the kidneys well and avoid the formation of stones and grit that can cause colic.

***

It helps to urinate also, the water of corn husks.

***

A real tonic that facilitates long and healthy urination is made as follows: boil parsley, corn husks, cane and grass. Drink the liquid and wait until you feel the urge to urinate, which will happen soon.

***

Drink infusions of horsetail. Drink Caribbean rum with mint water.

Drink infusions of blackthorn and cherry tail. Drink parsley decoctions.

***

Drink infusions of elderberry leaves, to which a glass of Scotch whisky has been added.

***

Drink infusions of birch leaves.

***

Or ash leaves, a product known since ancient times to be very diuretic.

***

The retention of urine is avoided by taking three cups a day, outside of meals, of parsnip infusion (Betula erecta).

***

The ingestion of infusions made with the bark of the root of díctamo, also known as fresnillo (Dictamnus albus), also avoids the retention of urine.

***

If the one who has problems urinating is a woman, take vapours of bird feathers, after burned, through the genitals.

To eliminate kidney stones

Against kidney colic, the very painful nephritic colic, apply dry heat in the area of the kidneys and drink many infusions of Arenaria (Herniaria glabra) until the stone is expelled or the kidneys are cleaned of stones.

***

Crumble an onion in white wine and add a broken radish, six grains of corn flour and a few drops of lemon. Cook it all. Drink the resulting liquid twenty-four hours later.

***

Sarsaparilla is also very good in juice or infusion.

**

Drink infusions of tostonera (Adiantum reniforme). It is a canary remedy.

**

Drink coclearia juice (Cochlearia officinalis). Drink infusions of ash leaves.

Drink thermal waters or mountain springs.

**

According to a very old recipe, to remove kidney stones take mallow leaves, cook with pink oil, remove from heat and add two or three egg whites, stir well and pour on a colored cloth or dirty wool, apply two or three times on the bladder. Or boil old watercress in wine, squeeze it, and apply it to the bladder.

Against kidney ailments

Crumble an onion in white wine and, breaking a radish and making flour with six grams of corn, pour a few drops of lemon over it. Then cook it all and drink it twenty-four hours later.

**

Take infusions of Lepidium leaves (Lepidiumlatifolium), both for kidney ailments and to facilitate urination.

**

Take infusions of Parietaria, which grows in the cracks of walls and on the banks of streams.

To prevent gonorrhea and other sex evils

The man should have half a lemon ready and, before intercourse, wet a finger with its juice. Introduce it into the woman's vagina and, if she feels itching or stinging, be rejected.

***

If there has been a suspicious sexual act, the man should go to a urinal or toilet. Squeeze the virile member strongly with one hand, below the acorn (or bud) and urinate. When the pressure is irresistible, squeeze the rest of the member with the other hand, pressing it with all your strength so that the urine will come out under pressure. Repeat the operation several times.

***

Drink arenaria in infusion, which favors the emission of urine because urinating a lot helps to get rid of infections.

***

In case of suspicious intercourse, or if any discomfort is noticed within twenty-four hours after intercourse, the man and the woman should wash their parts with infusions of chamomile, walnut, sarsaparilla, or mallow, which should also be drunk.

***

Wash the male member and vagina with raw lemon or orange juice.

***

Rub the member and vagina with onions cut in half, split garlic and parsley.

***

If gonorrhea is chronic, wash the affected parts with decoctions of marigold or marigold.

To cure sores of the anus or vulva

Apply to the affected areas, decoctions of the plant called bistorta (Polygonum bistorta).

***

Soak the lesions with decoctions of gorse or comfrey (Ajuga reptans), especially if the sore has degenerated into ulceration.

***

In general, for vaginal washes, practice these with walnut leaf decoctions.

To combat crabs

Give rubs of diesel oil all over the body, especially in the areas near the genitals. The woman should take special care so that the oil does not get into the vagina.

***

Shave the parts of the man or woman completely because crabs live among the hair of the genitals and wash them frequently.

Against impotence

The man should apply on the penis the powder resulting from shredding deer antlers.

***

To awaken sexual desire, oregano buds also seem to have been used.

***

To maintain erection, in some areas of Castile, men smeared their penis with the milky sap of some euphorbiaceae, such as the popularly called "lechi interna", actually the spurge (Euphorbia lathyris).

***

Method highly recommended nowadays, even by doctors, is to warm the penis with a very hot cloth until achieving the minimum erection necessary to proceed to penetration.

***

It is also not a bad system to introduce, pushing with his or her fingers the flaccid penis into the vagina because the natural heat of the feminine duct generally tends to straighten it.

***

Very traditional, and apparently quite widespread, was the belief that a miraculous method against impotence was the abundant ingestion of bull's testicles, that is to say, testicles of the aforementioned animal, conveniently prepared in stews with various vegetables.

***

A simpler remedy is to eat egg yolks every day, and even better if, for three consecutive days, the person concerned mixes such yolks with onion.

***

Very traditional seems to be also the belief that eating raw onion gives sexual potency to men and raw garlic. However, the best thing seems to be to intersperse onions, garlic and tomatoes, also raw, in the diet.

THE EXTREMITIES

However much work they throw at him, however many hours he has to sit at work, or however many leagues he has to endure on foot each day, it is necessary to take good care, however, both arms and legs, or upper and lower limbs, as you prefer, in addition to the concomitant parts that would say that Argentine healer, so that the foot never give a stumble ... And so that the hand does not walk on his ass, like the anus.

Against tremors of the fingers of the hands

Take barley decoctions.

From thigh to foot, or the problems of the legs

So far, nothing better has been found to relieve sore feet than to soak them in hot water with plenty of salt. The relief is immediate and very pleasant. So much so that in some Caribbean islands, it is also recommended even against male sexual impotence: "He who walks well, loves well", they say in the interior of the island of Puerto Rico. It is also good to take water from the sea and heat it up before putting your feet in it.

***

If the legs hurt, lie down on your side with the pillow between your thighs.

***

Ideal against leg pain, even if it is not rheumatic, is to put the patient's lower limbs in a basin, into which the viscera of a freshly slaughtered animal will have been poured.

***

For the pain of the knee, and in general that of the whole leg as well, take a bunch of each of the flowers and leaves that tradition knows as St. John's wort, which is the following: daisies (Chrysanthemum maximum), roses, elder leaves, ash and walnut. Let them boil in water, and the sick person sits on a chair so that the container is under his knees, which are covered with a blanket to receive the steam in the affected parts.

***

In general, and whenever possible, walk barefoot on the sand of the beach or along the shore of the same.

***

Immerse the sore feet in a pool where the sun has been shining, and you will instantly feel great relief.

***

If you want to wake up a sleeping foot without discomfort, make a cross with saliva on it.

Against rheumatism

Put dry heat on the joints. It is the best remedy known to relieve your pain.

***

Take thermal baths whenever possible. At home, the baths should be very hot water, as much as you can stand, throwing a lot of coarse salt in the bathtub.

***

Another good remedy consists in bathing the patient, for fifteen consecutive days, in a decoction of walnut and alder leaves, to which a kilo of salt should be added. It is also an excellent solution against lumbago.

***

Drink ferruginous waters.

*****

With the old ovens, which remain in the bakeries of some villages, you can follow a practice that greatly relieves rheumatics: make a big fire in the oven, then clean it and put the sick person there until the oven cools down.

*****

Rub the affected areas with nettles. This revitalizes the circulation.

*****

Rub the affected areas with alcohol or apple cider vinegar.

*****

Also excellent are the rubs with the peeled root of the black witch (Dioscorea communis), badger butter and Pyrenean dormouse fat.

*****

To take it, make a syrup made with sarsaparilla, rustic cumin (Margotia gummifera), heart flower or fumitory (Dicentra spectabilis) and guaiac (Guaiacum officinale). Boil everything for half an hour. Then remove from the fire, let it cool, and mix well with purple sugar and honey. Then put the mixture back on the fire. Finally, put it in a bottle and drink it twice a day. This is a Caribbean remedy.

*****

Take a five-eyed potato and put it in a bag, which should be kept in the sick person's clothes. As the potato softens, the rheumatic pains will disappear.

*****

Take a vapour of the decoction of bouquet flowers and laurel leaves.

*****

Apply poultices made with cooked rosemary leaves and red wine.

***

Or heat a handful of cabbage leaves and put them on the painful area.

***

Drink infusions of horsetail and juniper. The oil extracted from juniper berries was formerly used for this purpose and to combat gout.

Take vapours from boiling mallow leaves. Drink infusions of carrasquilla sticks.

***

Or infusions of mallow with a glass of garlic liqueur macerated in alcohol.

***

Eat garlic on an empty stomach or cook and drink its water. Rub yourselves with sugar cane rum.

***

Take infusions of elderflower and ground ivy mixed in equal parts. After each infusion, drink a short drink of Scotch whisky.

***

According to tradition, the fervor for Saint Eulalia greatly relieves the ills caused by rheumatism.

***

The magic tradition also commands to drink the water collected from the fountains on the morning of St. John.

***

Carry a potato in your pocket; better if it has been stolen from a villager. This remedy also comes from popular tradition.

**

Take sea baths; better if the water is artificially heated an odd number of times for nine consecutive days. This remedy was once very popular in some coastal areas.

**

Catch a live lizard with the iron of the oven. Fry it in boiling oil inside a covered casserole. After a while, add wine. Transfer everything to an earthenware pot and keep it there for twenty days. From then on, it can be rubbed on the painful region.

**

If all these remedies fail, you can still try to place on the painful area of the right foreleg of a hare, which according to some, always gives very good results.

Against arthrosis

Crush six cloves of garlic and half an onion in the juice of two lemons. Let it macerate in a liter of water overnight and take it in the morning for several days: it is one of the best natural remedies known against osteoarthritis, recommended by many doctors. Apply as a poultice.

**

Make a poultice with holly leaves, rice and garlic macerated in alcohol: put it hot on the area that hurts the most.

**

Make as much use of dry heat as necessary to relieve pain.

Against muscular injuries

Nothing better to relieve a muscle injury than the traditional hot water bottle.

To cure lumbago

Tie a thin matchstick candle around the patient's waist.

***

Give rubs with alcohol and nettles, alternately, on the lumbar area.

***

If nothing better is available, apply a hot espadrille or a hot brick to the painful region.

***

In some areas of France, they cure it by putting a little sugar on the kidneys of the patient.

***

According to the magic tradition, put on the kidneys of the sick person, the lilies spread during the Corpus Christi procession.

***

The lumbago is also cured if the sufferer wallows in the herbs of a meadow, better on the night of Saint John and naked.

***

A remedy from Extremadura consists of lying the patient face down on the ground, naked on his back, and being trampled by a barefoot twin.

Against sciatica

Tie a rope with nine knots around the painful leg and wear it until the pain disappears.

***

Rub warm oil on the lumbar area, which is then covered with a cloth. If you put a hot water bottle on top of it, the improvement comes almost immediately.

***

The patient should lie down on a bed of nettles.

Against hemiplegia

If the paralysis of half the body is stubborn, for nine days, the patient should drink a glass of freshly slaughtered pig's blood on an empty stomach, followed by half a small glass of rancid wine. Rest fifteen days and start again on the ninth until full recovery.

Against glandular eruptions

Rub the lesion with oil and milk cream.

***

To cure the golondrino or glandular infarction in the armpits or groin, in the morning, before sunrise, the patient being fasting, santiguase three times and squeeze the golondrino with three fingers of the hand in three different positions. Repeat the operation every day, taking care that there are three main feasts in succession between such days.

***

The remedy applied by the Basque healers is the following: make 81 crosses, with as many grains of wheat, over the lesions declaiming on each occasion the following psalm: "The swallows are nine; the nine † eight; the eight † seven; the seven † six; the six † five; the five † four; the four † three; the three † two; the two † one; the swallows are not one, may the Father, Son and Holy Spirit cure one". This operation is finished, record 81 Credos, after which the grains of wheat shall be thrown into the field for food for the birds. Apply the remedy three days in succession, and the lesions will disappear. Otherwise, it will be delayed as long as it takes to delay the cure.

THE NERVES

If your nerves are bad, you can lose them for any foolishness. Keeping them calm and appeased is as important as having a cool head or with good irrigation and without anguishing pains. As you know, with a stiff nerve, you risk losing your skin.

In order not to have bad nerves

The best thing to do is to drink infusions of lime blossom.

***

To calm a nervous person, squeeze an orange leaf between your fingers and put it under your nose so that he can smell it. He will soon calm down.

***

Take infusions of orange tree leaves and orange blossoms.

***

Every morning, bathe the nervous system with cold water.

***

A Caribbean remedy with proven effects consists of chewing tobacco.

***

Infusions of mint, marshmallow and lemon balm have a great calming effect.

***

Drink infusions of rosemary and horsetail. Ingest infusions of poppy.

***

According to tradition, drinking water on the morning of St. John's Day is preserved against nervous diseases.

**

Another traditional remedy: incinerate a live mole, pour its ashes in a bowl with water and add raw yarn, freshly spun. Cook, let it cool and drink it.

**

The Extremaduran tradition says that to be cured of a nervous attack, the affected person has to close himself in his room with a jackdaw and for three days feed himself only with the same food that the bird eats.

Against hysterism

Take infusions of the root of arcangelica. Two or three cups a day, but outside of meals.

**

Take gentian macerations. To do this, leave a piece of the plant in a coffee cup full of water for twenty-four hours, strain it after that time and drink the resulting liquid.

**

Especially if it is a woman who suffers from it, make her ingest rue oil.

**

It is also not bad to give the hysteric a couple of slaps.

**

But if that is too much, make the patient sneeze, and the hysteria will disappear.

Against startling

To avoid startles caused by an unforeseen fright, carry a few sprigs of rue between the person's clothes.

***

Valencian lands have been used to drink orange blossom water, an infusion of the same flower.

Against depression

Ingest infusions of mugwort from the Alps (Artemisia genipi). Two or three cups daily, but outside of meals, is recommended.

Against anxiety

Drink infusions of the plant called calamento (Calamintha sylvatica), mixed with lemon juice and a teaspoon of honey. The ideal is a cup on an empty stomach in the morning, another in the afternoon and another before going to sleep at night.

Against exhaustion

In addition to getting plenty of rest, drink juice of nasturtium leaves (Tropaeolum majus) mixed with milk or another aromatic product.

For sleep problems

To avoid insomnia, the affected person should pray to the saints to whom he/she is most devoted. The ideal is to repeat batches of rosaries.

***

Or, better still, drink an infusion of poppy petals before going to sleep.

***

Drink infusions of lemon balm.

Or hawthorn or hawthorn. Smell a chopped onion.

***

Apply a hedgehog fried in oil on the left eye of whoever suffers from insomnia, and he will sleep like a blessed.

***

In some places, to put a sleepless child to sleep, poppy seeds were placed under the pillow.

***

If you want to wake up at a specific time, and you are a believer, nothing is better than entrusting yourself to Saint Joseph.

***

Against nightmares, pray to any of these saints: Saint Agnes, Saint Andrew or Saint Mames naturally, if you are a believer. For the rest, they say, it is enough to wish fervently not to have bad dreams before going to bed.

For madness

Madness, because it has been considered since ancient times as a demonic evil, has had many magical and religious prescriptions, of dubious effect, however. But it is also known since the time of Maricastaña that some natural remedies can at least alleviate their ills.

***

Sea baths are a very good relaxing effect, especially when the waters are cold.

***

Rub the head of the sick person with violet and sweet almond oil.

***

Give the madman to drink goat's milk or the milk of a woman who has just given birth.

***

Let him who has suffered an attack of insanity ingest the brains of a black cat, and he will be cured of his ailment.

***

Give him an ounce of poppy syrup with rose water for him who does not sleep well because of the state of his mind.

Epilepsy and St. Vitus' Dance

These nervous ailments cause the sick person to convulse extraordinarily, so there is nothing better than the remedies described above for states of nervous excitement.

***

In addition, epileptic states are relieved by ingesting infusions of asperilla (Galium odoratum) moderately.

***

Also, with decoctions of primrose or primrose flowers (Primula vulgaris).

***

A similar effect is achieved by the patient eating the smoking heart of a snake.

***

Better yet, without the patient's knowledge, take a snake, step on its head and extract its heart. Said the reptile's heart, the epileptic will swallow it blindfolded.

***

Another remedy against epileptic seizures is to drink warm goat blood for three days in a row.

Or by swallowing the "bone" of a deer's heart.

***

A Galician remedy against epilepsy orders to burn the patient's shirt and make him eat part of the resulting powder. The same is used to alleviate menstrual pains for those who have them.

***

It was believed in several areas of Europe that epilepsy was cured by inhaling the dust resulting from crushing a human skull or the dust from the burnt bones of a person. The effect was reinforced if the deceased had been of the opposite sex to the sick person.

***

If the epileptic seizure has already occurred, make the affected person smell a sweaty and smelly shoe.

***

If what is wanted is to avoid having epilepsy, give the children, before suckling, water or wine in which a silver coin has been.

St. Vitus' dance is relieved by linden tea.

***

Both in the case of epilepsy and St. Vitus' dance, alcoholic beverages are contraindicated.

For the memory

It has been known since ancient times that eating pig's brains increases memory and prevents, with advancing age, the loss of memory that is common among the elderly.

***

89

As they say vulgarly, eating raisin tails is very good for keeping the memory fresh. And to review sentences. Of course, in reality, you can review anything that serves to give agility to the head. For example, the license plate numbers of the cars we see on the street. Or telephone numbers.

THE SKIN

Whoever's skin doesn't look good is a goner, because the skin, a good color, and a healthy appearance are our best business card for love, for work, and even to greet us day by day, happy and confident, without resentment against ourselves, in front of the mirror. For good skin, try to be as sweet as honey and do not make of your thoughts a compote of anger and gall, as the popular song says.

To avoid skin problems

Eat raw snake meat in abundance.

To put an end to any problem of the epidermis

Give the patient a daily walk around a rose bush for nine consecutive days, saying: "The rose with the roses". To reinforce the remedy, on the ninth day, he should go around the same rose bush nine times in a row.

***

If what is wanted is to end an inflammation of the skin, apply to the patient poultices of cornmeal on the affected area.

To eliminate the skin eruption

Rub the diseased part with the blood of three roosters' crests belonging to three different houses. None of the three roosters should be from the patient's own house.

***

The patient should be carried a long way on his back by another person who, having suffered from the same disease, managed to be cured.

Against infantile dermatitis

Mix olive oil with well-beaten egg white and apply to the affected area.

Against juvenile acne

When it presents purulent scabs, take borage infusions out of meals.

***

It is also good to take infusions of dandelion roots and leaves.

***

Pick elderflowers on the morning of St. John's Day, cook them in a cauldron and let them cool. Then wash your face with it for all the members of the family.

***

Wet your face with alcohol diluted with water.

To get rid of warts

As annoying as they are ugly and with the danger of becoming something worse than a wart, especially if they bleed or come out in soft parts such as the armpits, genital area and groin, warts are nevertheless well treated by natural methods. According to some magical traditions, for example, in the Caribbean and the Canary Islands, warts appear to those who look at the stars at night for a long time, and the best way to cure them is to go to sleep early and not look at the sky, which punishes those who do not go to bed.

***

The healer personally counts warts on the wart, without forgetting neither the smallest nor the most hidden of the whole body, and retains the number in memory or writes it down. Send the patient home and wait for the healer until it is dark. Then go to a mill and dip the hand in the water at the entrance. If the number of warts is even, do this with the moon in crescent and with the hand in the water, say three Hail Marys. If the number of warts is odd, on the contrary, do the operation with the moon is waning and pray only two Hail Marys. Think that a mistake in counting, even the smallest, makes this therapy ineffective.

***

But, apart from magical traditions, we have found that to cure warts, it is very useful to take an early fig, cut it and pass the juice over the wart. Of course, a fig should be used for each wart.

***

Another good remedy is to remove the milk from a handful of early figs and rub it carefully on warts until it is absorbed.

***

According to another magical tradition, if you take as many salt stones as warts you want to cure and throw them on the road without looking back, warts you have will stick to the first person who passes by.

***

Kill a lizard and prick it with a pin, as many times as warts the wart you want to cure has. Keep the animal in a jar, cover it, and when it has dried, warts will also have dried. It is a remedy of the Valencian healers.

***

It is also said that by making a cross with jonquils and burying it immediately after, and if you then say any prayers, warts disappear from where the affected person has them.

**

Likewise, the rush is used in the following remedy. Pluck several rushes from the ground by the affected person, but with his hands crossed behind his body so that he cannot see the plants at the moment of plucking them. Then pass the rushes over warts, tracing crosses over them and placing them on the chimney so they may dry soon.

**

In any case, it is much more effective to drink water in which wheat has been boiled. If this is done at least once every day, warts will disappear sooner rather than later.

**

Take as many grains of wheat as there are warts on the wart and rub the corresponding lesion with each of them. Hide the grains of cereal under a stone, and, when they have been corrupted, warts will be cured.

**

Rub them with a coin, put them inside an envelope and leave it at a crossroads. Whoever picks up the envelope will be loaded with warts, and whoever leaves it will be free of them.

**

A good recipe is to cut an apple into four pieces and rub warts with its flesh. Tradition dictates to bury the pieces of the apple immediately, and better without the person concerned knowing the place. Do it to whoever considers it best. Others prefer to practice this remedy with potatoes.

**

The goodness of this remedy has been demonstrated: eat a lime, then rub it on warts. It is also said that the effect is faster if the slime or slug is buried in a crack in the wall.

***

Rub the lesions with slime or slug and then nail the animal behind the door of the house. As it dries, warts will also dry. It is necessary not to wash the affected area for several days. The slug will remain on the door until, by touching it with your fingers, it falls apart.

***

Wash warts with the warm blood of a freshly killed bull.

***

The best of all: rub warts with split and oozing garlic. Tradition dictates that the garlic be placed on the hearth for three Fridays.

The tradition says to put the garlic on the fire for three Fridays: this is the time it takes for the remedy to take effect.

***

It is also good to rub warts with a piece of fresh meat, which logically should not be eaten later: it is necessary to throw it away, although some traditions command to let it rot in sight. The truth is that in the time it takes for the piece of meat to rot, warts rubbed with it will disappear.

***

Equally good or better results are obtained by rubbing warts with a piece of fresh bacon.

***

In some areas, the warts are rubbed with open potatoes. This is the most effective remedy in hot areas. In the Caribbean, the same is done with raw plantain.

***

Dip a crumb of bread in common vinegar, put the crumb on the wart and cover it with a plaster. This should be done as many days as necessary until the wart disappears.

***

Formerly the warts were pricked with a hot needle, but for that, it is preferable to go to a skin doctor.

***

A remedy as simple as rubbing warts with a woman's menstrual blood is also no longer used, and yet it seemed to give very good results. A drop was smeared on each lesion, morning and evening, for several days. If a menstruating woman was not at hand, mole's blood also served as a substitute.

***

Nor was there a Basque method of a magical nature, as simple as the warty person going to mass and, when the officiant said the Orate Frates, the affected person would answer Kanpora -Fuera-verrugates.

To eliminate pimples in general

They disfigure the face of the young and worry everyone. A good remedy is washing your face in the morning with raw lemon and letting it dry. After a while, wash your face again with water.

***

To eliminate common pimples, soak your face with hot water and salt.

Apply the blood purifying remedies already mentioned above. Garlic, onions and lemon are magnificent.

Put on them a good piece of roasted onion.

***

To eliminate pimples around the waist.

Someone who has had them before cut a rooster's crest and rubbed the patient's pimples with its blood. While the operation is being performed, the patient should remain half-naked on the floor. At the end of the therapy, incorporate the patient and go to a crossroads, where he will pray for nine Our Fathers for the one who applied the remedy. Not only will he be healed, but from that moment on, he will be endowed with the virtue of healing others.

***

It is still a belief, but if you do the lemon, garlic and onions, it will surely give better results.

Against eczema

Rub the lesion with honeysuckle.

Against urticaria

Drink infusions of Calophyllum (Geum urbanum) mixed with a teaspoon of honey, and no more than three a day.

***

Rub with holy water the body of those who suffer from it. Italians and French say that there is no better remedy against urticaria.

Against boils and boils

The same applies to pimples, but as they are more stubborn, it is advisable to treat them more carefully. Thus, put on the area of a poultice made with St. John's wort.

***

Another proven remedy consists of crushing a snail in the hands and rubbing the boils with everything that results from it: they dry in a very short time.

***

In the Canary Islands, they used to apply the mud with water on the lesion as a poultice, holding it afterwards with a bandage. The same has been done with chewed wheat and even with a piece of tomato. After ten to thirty minutes, the pus would be released.

Take infusions of horsetail.

***

Soak absorbent cotton in horsetail infusion and wipe the boil.

***

Rub with an open onion, with oil or with brandy.

***

Fry elder bark in olive oil over low heat. When the juice oozes out, remove the remaining liquid from the pan and add to the remaining virgin wax. Let it cool, and put it on the boils when the mass is solid.

***

Mix the yolks of nine hard-boiled eggs, nine drops of wine, nine drops of oil, nine drops of honey and nine drops of fennel root. Pass it all through a sieve and take it to the sick person. It is a Saxon remedy.

***

Rub with onion and oil or with onion and soap. Ingest infusions of walnut leaves and bark.

***

Or burdock or burdock (Arctium lappa) is also an excellent blood purifier.

***

Apply warm poultices of brewer's yeast to the affected area.

Against erysipelas

Wash the affected area with mallow and plantain water. Then apply with absorbent cotton the juice of blackberry herb (Solanum nigrum), or hot honey, and bandage.

***

Pour some wine, oil, salt and water into an earthenware bowl, then make a swab of unwashed wool and, soaked in this mixture, anoint the diseased area.

***

Take a black hen, shake it alive and place it on the head of the sick person. It is a Basque remedy from Alava.

Drink the affected person the blood of a male hare or lizard.

***

Although the simplest remedy is undoubtedly chewing esparto grass, or freshly sprouted fern, with the teeth.

Against herpes

The simplest procedure is to rub it with saliva on an empty stomach.

***

Or with the urine of a black cat.

***

For more problematic cases, drink a glass of sulphurous water twice daily. Failing that, add 300 grams of white honey and 75 grams of burdock (Arctium lappa) to the fountain's water and administer one spoonful in the morning and one in the evening.

***

A Central American tradition commands a virgin girl to urinate on the herpes of the affected person.

***

Prepare an ointment by mixing garlic and esparto ashes and oil, wet it with a live bird feather, and spread it on the affected part of the patient.

***

Whoever suffers from this affection takes on his back another person who has suffered from the same, and with him on his back, walks around a table seven times.

***

Catch a snake, skin it and clean it well. Then crumble a piece of it and season it into an omelette. Give it to the patient to eat.

***

Mix ashes from a campfire and water, and soak several strips of white cloth with the resulting mass. Apply overnight to the affected part, fasten it with a bandage, and remove in the morning.

***

It is also convenient here to use the blood depurative, previously mentioned in its corresponding section.

Against anthrax

Place a live toad on the pimple, fastened with a bandage, and keep it there until the animal dies, which usually happens after about eight days, and the carbuncle will be cured.

Against scrofula

Rub with unsalted butter.

***

Pick esparto flowers on the morning of St. John's Day before sunrise. Let the esparto flower dry. Then throw the flowers on the embers and heat in the smoke a cloth that will then be placed on the lesions.

***

Magical tradition dictates that the scrofula be rubbed with a coin, which is then wrapped with five grains of corn in a piece of cloth.

The magical tradition commands to rub the scrofula with a coin, then wrap it with five grains of corn in a piece of paper and throw it all at a crossroads.

***

However, in this second case, it offers better results to gently rub the scrofula lumps with grains of salt, or with laurel leaves, with a little more energy.

***

Ingest decoctions of red nettle.

***

Take gentian macerations. We explained how to prepare them when referring to hysterism.

***

In the past, scrofula was cured in some regions of England by simply having a fasting virgin touch it.

Against sebaceous cysts

Pass a chickpea 100 times over the cyst, scratching it at the same time, always following the direction of the tendon.

To cure corns

It is said that cutting off the tip of the callus can cure them.

***

Soak your feet in warm water and rub the corns with a pumice stone.

***

Apply a hot potato to them often.

***

To soften them, soak your feet in hot water with salt or soap, and rub the calluses with a brush.

***

To cure corns, take some wrapping paper, soak it with vinegar and place the patient in a saucer under the bed. It is a southern European remedy.

***

Corns are also cured with saliva on an empty stomach or by dissolving an oyster pearl in lemon juice and soaking the lesion with it at night. It is another southern European remedy.

Against scabies

From ancient times it has been believed that drinking milk and eating fritada on the first day of May cures scabies. It is another tradition.

***

It works well to crush the root of Colchicum autumnale (Colchicum autumnale) mixed with salt and the patient's own urine. Rub it all over the affected area before going to bed.

***

Wash the patient twice a day, for two consecutive days, with sulfur water and nettles. On the third day, the disease should be cured. If not, repeat the operation until necessary.

***

Rub the whole body of the affected person with lard and sulfur, and stay by the fire.

***

It was believed that to cure scabies, it was good to go naked to the field on the morning of St. John, before dawn, to absorb the dew of the sunrise.

To absorb the dew of dawn.

***

Rub the scabies lesions with pulverized eggshell.

***

In some places of Central America and the Caribbean, the tradition commands to kiss the snout of seven dogs that wander in the street, pass them the mange and clean the sick person.

***

A Navarrese remedy recommends that, if a child suffers from scabies, a woman should take the patient in her arms while fasting and take him to where there is a wild rose bush. With the child in her arms, she will go around the bush three times, at the same time, also three times, repeating: "Scabies, to the rose". Once the operation is finished, the woman has to pray an Our Father. The operation should be repeated a few days later if the child is not cured.

Against ringworm

Apply the ringworm on the affected part, decoctions of burdock or burdock (Arctium lappa).

Against leprosy

Eat the affected person's fried snake in abundance.

***

The leper should be wrapped in stubble or herbs on the night of St. John, preferably at midnight on the dot.

***

Impregnate the affected person with the urine of a strong and healthy boy.

To kill nits and lice

Coat the hair with oil and drag the parasites with a comb. Catch and destroy them manually with the edge of the nails.

Apply oil to the affected person's head.

***

Rub the head, whoever needs it, with fine powder from the earth of an orchard.

To make chilblains disappear

Soak in baths of hot and cold water, alternately.

***

They are cured very well by rubbing them with garlic and verbena.

***

Rub with strawberries on the affected area or with a clove of garlic.

**

Urinate them on the affected person as soon as he/she gets up in the morning.

**

Rub nettles on the chilblains and then urinate them on the affected person.

**

Immerse the affected limbs in hot water used to boil chestnuts.

**

Although it seems more effective to heat some iron tongs on the fire, to rub each chilblain three times with them, you can vary the number of rubs, but it is essential, for the remedy to take effect, that it is always odd and does not exceed nine times.

**

According to some peasants of Monte, near Santander, to cure chilblains, there is nothing better than rubbing them on the intimate parts of a woman who has not washed them. They claim to have verified the goodness of this remedy.

INFECTIONS

If you want to live a lot, avoid the pus as when you don't have quarters, you avoid the game of mus. Or, what comes to the same thing, protect yourself against infections, whatever they are, making use of what is expressed to prevent and cure them. Fight infection, and you will be strong as a lion!

To avoid contagion

To present oneself smoking before a contagious patient avoids the contagion, especially if the smoked thing is a cigar. It is a very old and widespread popular belief.

***

Whoever appears before a contagiously sick person, in general, should do it carrying a piece of raw garlic in the nostrils of each nostril.

***

To avoid the contagion of smallpox, whoever takes care of a sick person who has brought such disease, should insert a clove of garlic in each nostril to avoid contagion through the breath. Also, note the precaution of tying as many heads of this product to the wrists to prevent the disease from entering the blood through the skin.

To improve the air in a room

Have in it a geranium flower.

***

Burn dry laurel leaves in a pan. It is also a good remedy against constipation.

Against localized infections

Apply an ointment, prepared as follows: take a few pieces of elder bark, remove the outer layers and, cut into small thin pieces, fry in a pan over low heat with olive oil. When all the juice has oozed out, remove it from the pan and add a little virgin wax to the remaining liquid. Place in a jar or similar container, and when it has cooled and solidified, it will be ready for use.

***

Another poultice to cure infections is prepared with the following ingredients: the tallow of a cow's kidney, 400 grams of lard, 500 grams of resin, 500 grams of virgin wax, a liter of olive oil, and a kilo and a half of chicken grass (Sedum telephium). The tallow, the lard and the resin should be cut into small portions, as well as the medicinal plants, including the leaves and stems. Put all this in a large pot on the fire. When it comes to a boil, let it simmer until all the ingredients, including the herbs, are completely melted. Then filter and squeeze through a bleached cloth with bleach, and place in a tureen, while the contents are still clean, with plastic wrap, and tie with string. The product will acquire a hard and oily consistency and brownish color when it has cooled. It can be prepared at any time of the year. Apply on the affected area with a piece of a sheet previously washed with bleach, fold and put on the fire to melt enough. Place a compress or absorbent cotton on top and bandage. Renew the cure every twenty-four hours or twice a day if the lesion oozes.

***

If nothing better is available, apply water in which garlic has been boiled on the affected part.

Against cholera

The same as against strong diarrhea: drink pure lemon juice in large quantities.

***

Or eat a lot of garlic and onions.

Against typhus

A recommendation against typhus, which has given very good results in the past, is to drink a glass of fresh sweetened water on an empty stomach for forty days in a row.

***

It was formerly believed that figs were harmful and that they could transmit the typhus disease since it was observed that it tended to develop

It was observed that the disease tended to develop in September and October when figs ripen, but there does not seem to be any connection between the two.

***

The best natural remedy against typhus, if we look at the abundant evidence we have of its goodness, consists in placing a large bucket of boiling water, putting a chair in the center of the bucket, sitting the sick person naked in it, and, although he has a high fever and diarrhea, covering him with a blanket. When the sick person sweats more because of the heat and fever, take him out of there and put him in a tub of cold water. Take him out soon after, and the next day he will experience a clear improvement. The most normal thing is that some tumors sprout in the back and in the legs, which will open spontaneously soon after expelling a dark liquid, like blood, with which the disease will go away.

When measles is present

Wash the patient's whole body with a decoction of mallow or wheat bran flour.

***

Wash the patient's eyes with salted water.

***

Keep the patient under the bed mattress. This treatment is also suitable for cases of smallpox.

***

Indistinctly for patients with smallpox or measles, they should remain wrapped in red sackcloth. The therapy will be reinforced if there is only one light, red, in the room where they are.

***

Give the sick person to drink infusions of elderflower, very sweetened.

Against scarlet fever

If some hairs are cut from the patient's head and fed to a donkey, mixed with his usual food, it will be the animal who will carry the disease.

Against fever

Choose, or combine, any of the following procedures: ingest one or several glasses of punch, rub the body strongly with nettles or introduce the patient to a bathtub or other container with cold water.

***

Rub the patient's legs from the knees down with hot water mixed with ashes.

***

Drink infusions of nettle stalks.

***

If a nursing infant suffers from it, put on socks moistened with vinegar.

***

In the case of a very high fever, a remedy to wrap the patient with a sheet soaked in cold water was not disdained in the past.

***

It is also very good to ingest decoctions of argáfita, thyme, rue, a type of fern known as tostonera canaria (Adiantum reniforme) and siempreviva (Gomphrena perennis), not as an aphrodisiac but for fever. It is a canary remedy.

***

Ideal for applying mustard poultices on the soles of the feet.

***

Put a frog in a cardboard box, put it on the navel of the afflicted person, tying the box with a bandage or with adhesive tape sold in pharmacies, leaving the whole thing there for two hours. Repeat the operation morning, afternoon and night. The frogs die with the heat of the fever they absorb, and the sick person heals.

Put raw and open potatoes on the forehead.

***

Or burn eucalyptus or laurels in the house when someone suffers from fever. It is also good for the flu.

***

Put three cloves of crushed garlic in a cloth with pork fat boiled in vinegar. This paste is then rubbed on the chest of the feverish person. It is also good against influenza and pneumonia, which cause a high fever.

***

Give the patient cold water baths, and make him drink many glasses of water, keeping him warm if it is cold weather or naked if it is hot.

***

Fennel herbal teas and the application of water and oil enemas are also excellent.

***

Drink infusions of borage.

***

Drink decoctions of pulverized elderberry bark.

***

The ideal is also the marshmallow root decoctions and ingesting red asphodel seeds (Asphodedus fistulous).

***

Chest massages with salted butter are very useful.

***

If, in addition to fever, the patient has chilled, rub the chest and back with nettles.

***

Or rub the patient's whole body with garlic and put a hot brick on his feet.

***

In the case of a dying patient in a feverish state, open a live rabbit in a carcass and place it on the head of the patient as a cap.

***

If the intention is to be preserved from fever for a whole year, tie the person's left arm to a tree before dawn, pray three Our Fathers and three Hail Marys, and then remove the arm, leaving the ligature behind the tree. This way, possible fevers will attack the tree, not the person.

Against tertian fevers

Drink a glass of wine to which the dust from filing the nails has been added. In Puerto Rico, nail powder is considered an aphrodisiac and is used in drinks, preferably alcoholic, before sexual intercourse or coitus.

***

The patient should drink the urine of a virgin woman or a child. The same remedy is used against jaundice.

***

Whoever suffers from tertian or quartan fevers, take a wand, better if it is of oleander, and go out at dawn to a crossroads of roads that no one has passed before him that day. Draw a cross on the ground with the wand and say: "Calenturas I bring, / Calenturas I have. / Who buys them for me? / I don't want them!" Then throw down the wand and run away without looking back. Whoever picks up the wand will henceforth bear the calenturas. It is assumed that the remedy will be strengthened if the bark of the oleander wand is cut nine times and grouped in threes.

***

Get out of bed at midnight and, in the dark and groping, go to the well of his house or the neighbour's, and throw a handful of salt previously provided. When throwing it, say the following: "San Crispinito, / San Crispinón, / tercianas I bring, / tercianas they are. / Here I leave them to you / that I don't want them". Return to your bedroom the same way as when you left, but without looking back and stepping where you stepped before. Repeat the operation three consecutive nights.

***

Knead a cake with olive oil, place it for a long time under the armpit, and feed it to the dogs. The animals will catch the fever, but he will be cured.

***

Let the patient with fever go to bed thinking about his illness without exchanging a word with anyone during the whole night. After one o'clock in the morning of the day, the fever does not correspond to him, and before dawn, he gets up and goes out to the field in search of a bush, trying not to meet anyone or, if that happens, refraining from greeting him. Once in front of the bush, he will respectfully uncover his head, if he is wearing a hat, cap or beret, and his coat, cloak or pinch, and he will say with fervor: "God keeps you, blackberry, / Come to God at this hour.

/ I come to you for a garment / of your whitish-green leaves, / for no one like you / can give me the salt". After saying this, take as many leaves from the bramble bush as you have suffered from hot flashes, taking care that they are nones, and return home by a different route than the one used to come, with the back of the hand where the leaves are resting on your back, praying a Creed for each leaf and releasing them one by one afterwards, without, for anything in the world, looking back.

POISONINGS AND BITES

From bad bugs, free yourself from your own hand, or what is the same, when an animal bites you, go quickly to apply to yourself what you are reminded here, because if you do not do it, perhaps you will rot and end up more screwed up than a whore in stubble or a dog on ice, downhill and without skates.

Against poison in general

Until you receive first aid, or if nothing better is available, drink plenty of raw milk.

***

Put seven cloves of garlic in a container with water that fits in a glass. Boil everything until its volume is reduced by half. Drink the resulting liquid on an empty stomach. This remedy is ideal against poisoning caused by animals.

Against rabies

According to an ancient tradition, garlic sown on Christmas day and harvested on St. John's day have the same virtue against rabies as the bread of Christmas Eve.

***

The truth is that garlic is a good remedy against rabies or hydrophobia, taken raw or rubbed on the chest and neck of those who a rabid dog has bitten.

***

Drink water with salt. The same should be given to rabid dogs.

***

Take the affected person on an empty stomach for nine consecutive days, nine teaspoons of the following preparation: in a pot, boil in beer six ounces of crushed rue, to which garlic, triain and tin scrapings are added.

***

When presented with a person bitten by a rabid dog, have the salutatorian fry oil and smear the wound with his fingers. The patient will feel pain, but the greeter, on the contrary, not the slightest. Then blow on the bite and a piece of bread, which the patient will have to eat.

Against dog bites

An ancient remedy commands to cure the bite of a dog or any other animal by putting on the wound hairs of the aggressor's tail.

***

In case of a bite, eat a lot of raw garlic immediately to purify the blood. Tradition tells the case of a young man, bitten by a rabid dog, who his parents locked in the kitchen of the house with the intention of leaving him there until he was cured. It did not take him long to come out, as he ate a couple of strings of garlic that were hanging on the wall and was cured. The same tradition warns that the garlic must have been sown on Christmas Eve and picked before sunrise on St. John's Day.

***

Take a mouthful of hot oil and gargle without swallowing it. Then spit the oil on the bite of the animal.

***

Put boiled nettles, and once softened, place them on the bite, pressing them with a handkerchief or a cloth.

***

Or rub the area of the bite with garlic or cut it into small slices and apply it to the wound, covering it with a bandage.

***

Or rub the bite with a mixture made, in equal parts, of fish glue and alum, all melted in natural vinegar.

For viper bites

Very good are the alder bark plasters.

***

Take a knife and make two cuts in the bite so that the venom bleeds. Put the wounded part in the water of a river without taking it out for at least half an hour.

***

Put on the bite of the viper the anus of a live chicken, which will act as a suction cup extracting the venom.

***

Apply a poultice of garlic, oil and ash tree roots to the bite.

***

Cover the bite with ox excrement or cow dung. After half an hour, wash the wounded part very well.

For snake bites

If you manage to kill the snake, cut off three fingers of its tail and rub the bite with it. The same effect is obtained if you rub the wound with the crushed head of the reptile.

***

Remove the wound with a knife and extract as much blood as possible.

***

Sprinkle the wound with a very crushed glass of a black bottle.

***

Drink mallow water. Then soften a tobacco leaf in strong brandy and put.it on the wound. Add a piece of plantain crumbled in a mortar. Then give the bitten person the resulting liquid to drink.

***

Immediately after the bite, record twenty Salves, numbering them one by one in a loud voice. Then apply a poultice with a lot of garlic, warm oil, ash root, poppy and Scrophularia. Cover it all with ox excrement and fasten it with a cloth. It will be observed that it will soon begin to purge the wound.

***

When the healer presents himself before the bitten person, pray the following: "Oh Mary, I offer you seven salves in the name of..." - here, he will say the name of the patient-. Recite these salves making the sign of the cross at the beginning and at the end of the fifth and seventh salves. Repeat the operation at the same time the next day, but make the second cross at the end of the fourth Salve. Do the same on the third day as on the first. Each day, at the end of the prayers, apply a poultice of oil, garlic and ash roots to the wound.

***

Pray immediately, without interruption or distraction, the Creed in reverse.

Against insect bites

To avoid them, rub the body with fresh leaves of wormwood, known in many places as absinthe (Artemisia absinthium), black horehound (Ballota nigra) or blackberry (Solanum nigrum).

***

Put cold fomentations of water, alcohol, ammonia or vinegar on the bites.

***

If the sting is a bee sting, extract the sting and make the wound bleed.

***

If stung by the same animal, rub the lesion with fresh leeks; better if it is with the white part of them.

***

It is very good, both for wasp stings and bee stings, to urinate on the stung area.

***

Or smear the lesion with garlic mashed in honey. First, apply the garlic and then the honey.

***

Put on the wound water with bleach.

***

If nothing better is available, rub the bite with the earth.

Against scorpion bites

Catch the animal, chop it into very small pieces and apply on the bite.

***

If the animal manages to escape, bite or cut off some of the skin of the sting and suck until all the venom is extracted.

***

Another remedy, if the scorpion has not been caught, is to place a piece of pig skin over the wound.

***

Put embers on a plate, add a few drops of olive oil and smoke the sting with everything.

***

In many places where there are scorpions, they are usually trapped and boiled in oil. With this oil, scorpion stings can be cured and those of spiders, bees and other insects, in addition to relieving the most varied pains. Several decades ago, we met a healer from Guadix (Granada), a great expert in the elaboration of scorpion oil, with a secret formula known only to him, which, when applied in the form of butter, even served to alleviate certain ailments of the female sex.

Against fish bites

Whoever pokes himself with a fish bone, dip the affected part in ammonia. Then hit the place where the thorn is lodged with a stick to extract it or expel as much blood as possible. Complete the treatment by ingesting seawater.

***

Or bleed the affected limb or immerse it in water with bleach.

For sea spider bites

Cauterize the affected area with a hot iron.

***

Remove the black slime left by the bite with the tip of a knife and scrape the area with a goat horn.

Against nettle stings

An infallible remedy so that nettles do not sting, and very simple, by the way, consists of holding your breath when they are to be touched, pulled out or manipulated.

***

But if, in spite of this precaution, you end up being stung, rub the affected area with mint.

THE TRAUMATISMS

If a blow hits you, take care of yourself soon and do not be a sledgehammer, because not having ideas or resources is sometimes bad, since you are left broken, fané and descangallado, as a famous tango says. There are so many things to be cured within these cases that not to do it more than abandonment; it is the incuriousness of a fool, the stubbornness of a mental cripple.

To avoid accidents when jumping

Before jumping, say to yourself: "I jump, I jump, from a haystack; if I break my head, God will cure it".

***

Or take the necessary precautions because, as you know: "A Dios rogando, pero con el mazo dando", as the popular saying goes. Or, what is the same: Pray, but do not stop rowing.

Against localized inflammations

Beat wine, oil and sugar and apply the resulting mixture, with a cotton ball, to the affected area.

***

Bathe the injured region with boiled water with salt, applying at the same time vigorous massages.

Against torticollis

When the affected person takes off his socks or stockings, leave the one corresponding to the left foot turned inside out or inside out before going to bed.

***

Rub the painful part with a piece of very hot red wool. Against haemorrhages from wounds

Apply soot and burnt cloth sparks on the wound.

***

Put the wound under a stream of cold water.

***

If the wound is not very considerable, apply directly to it spider's web.

***

If the wound occurs on the high seas and nothing better is at hand, burn it with wine and brandy and cover it with a handkerchief.

If even this is not available, urinate on it.

***

For haemorrhages, it is also very good to apply ice to the wound.

***

Although it is said that the best thing to do is undoubtedly to lick it with a dog, which will remove the bad blood from the patient's body; however, it has been believed that the animal would end up contracting rabies.

For a wound to heal well

Cover with fat without salt, on which a leaf of those that are raised in the brambles near the streams has to be placed. Failing that, a fig leaf can be used. It is necessary to avoid, for the treatment to be effective, the proximity of the sea.

***

For a wound to heal well, wash it with water in which garlic has been boiled. Add a few drops of lemon. Apply mercurochrome and a lettuce leaf smeared with the same product on it. Fasten it all with a dressing or bandage.

***

So that a wound does not occur again in the place where there was another smear, the first with the gizzard of a kid still hot and, in turn, heated on the fire.

Against infected wounds

The procedure known as marker water consists of boiling water in an earthenware pot filled almost to the brim. Put three bay leaves and twelve white pebbles, the so-called salt abundant on the banks of streams and streams. When the water is boiling, it is poured into a wide clay pot, in the center of which the pot will be placed upside down, avoiding that the stones and the leaves of laurel come out. On the bottom of the pot, place a pair of scissors, a knife and a crossed comb. Over all this, keep the affected limb covered with a cloth for about ten minutes. The operation should be repeated until healing is achieved. Some have been used to add to the boiling water nine small pieces of tile and even a few garlic. If the treatment fails, resort to the decoction of rose centifolia or one hundred leaves or to the poultice prepared with a liter of vinegar and a quart of powder.

***

It is also good to squeeze drops of celandine sap directly into the infected lesion.

***

If a wound is ulcerated, cover it with honey and wrap it with a bandage.

To heal any wound or graze, infected or not

Fry ten heads of garlic in half a pound of oil, which must be removed when it comes to a boil. Then add six ounces of virgin wax and minium powder. The resulting black ointment is ready for use when the wax has melted. Apply directly to the affected spot. Keep the excess in a tin can.

To cure sores

Wash the lesions with water in which rosemary has been boiled.

***

Or with decoctions of bistorta (Polygonum bistorta).

Against bruises

Place a piece of brown paper on the bruise, moistened and sprinkled with sugar, and soon positive effects will be observed.

To treat gangrene

Wash the affected area with nettle infusions.

***

Or of clavelina de Marte, also known in some areas as the "herb of ulcers".

***

If the disease was internal, leeches were once applied to remove the corrupted blood.

Against sprains

Everyone has them from time to time, so we all know how painful they are. Formerly it was believed that menstruating women suffered more from them because of a supposed weakness in their limbs, but now we know better. Anyone can suffer a sprain, even if they do not run or play sports. It is enough to carelessly go up or down the curb.

***

For the magical tradition, the sprain was cured by joining the separated parts, for which it was recommended to take a sewing needle that would have to go three times through a loose thread in some fabric.

***

It was also recommended to give the injured person as many frictions on the painful area as he/she had for years. And fold a clean apron over the sore limb; someone would say the Creed backwards or some other prayer, and then the patient was to turn a walnut tree three times around and around.

Was to turn a walnut tree three times, from left to right.

***

Another of the oldest traditions commands to put a few coals of fire in a pot. From the herbs blessed on St. John's Day, a few small balls are made, which are thrown five times into the fire, saying each time while exposing the painful area to the smoke: "By virtue of the Holy Spirit, be healed".

***

However, it seems more effective to put on the affected area a poultice made with wheat bran flour, eggs and wine.

***

Apply arnica poultices on the affected area. They can be painful until you get used to them, but they are excellent for combating the pain caused by a sprain, a blow or any contusion.

***

Against the blows, massage with unsalted butter on the affected area.

***

Spread warm honey on the affected part and bandage.

***

As soccer players do, hold an ice pack on the sore part. Afterwards, go to the bone setter or petriquillo, or keep absolute rest.

***

It is not advisable to drink milk during the days in which rest is kept by a sprain injury, to avoid the accumulation of uric acid.

***

Massage with olive oil and mint macerated in it, the affected part.

***

Put warm red wine cloths over the injury, as the tannin in the wine reabsorbs the inflammation. Mulled wine cloths, by the way, are a very good remedy also for muscular pain in the neck and back.

***

Let us look at a famous Basque method to reduce a sprain. In case the patient has a sprained ankle, the healer begins by reciting: "Holy glorious Agueda, give me the grace to return the bones and flesh to their place". Take then between his fingers about 10 centimeters of beret strip and with it make nine crosses at different points of the affected area, rhythmically reciting the following formula: "Vein tractioned, vein injured, vein get into your place". Then recite three Our Fathers and three Hail Marys. Finally, place a cloth soaked in oil and wine over the affected area and order the affected person to rest absolutely, keeping the foot stretched out and supported on a stool or chair. Repeat the operation for three consecutive days. If there is no improvement, heat sea water, soak a cloth and apply it to the lesion. Although drinking water with salt is useful, it is less effective.

To cure a sprain

If it is a sprained foot, look for a widow offering a simple cure. But it must be a serious woman, and those who do not meet this requirement are useless. Once this is done, place the injured foot on the ground, pass the widow over it three times, rest her heel, and turn it by pressing it down with force. You should not be frightened or be softened by the patient's cries. Otherwise, the method will have no effect.

To cure dislocations and strains

Approach the affected person to a fountain that never dries out and picks up nine pebbles. With each one of them, make a cross on the affected point and recite: "These stones and these bones, / return to their place, / as the water of this fountain prial / ran to the sea". It is an Asturian remedy.

***

The curandera or curandero gathers nine stones, taken from the goterales of a hórreo -the ones from a breadbasket or six-legged hórreo are not useful-. Take one of the stones and trace a semicircle over the affected part, from top to bottom and then in reverse, and recite: "Corda saltada, / corda cabalgada, / que na carne fuege criada, / da carne pasáchete al hoso; / vólvete al tou llugar, / como Jesucristo al sou altar". Repeat the operation with each stone for three days. This is another Asturian remedy.

***

If it is a question of reducing muscular distension, give the healer a good massage on the affected part of the patient. Then place it on a pot where mistletoe leaves have been cooked, so it receives the mist. Dress the injured region properly and lay the patient well wrapped up so that he sweats.

***

To cure the same problem, thread the healer in a needle and unknotted strand of the patient's garment. It should be a sock, regardless of the part of the body where the distension has occurred, as this will have a greater healing effect. Pass this thread through the garment an odd number of times and say at the same time to the healer: "Stretched tendon, torn tendon, the tendon goes into place". Finish the operation with the recitation of an Our Father and Hail Mary, or a Creed. For best results, pray these prayers backwards and forwards. It also reinforces the therapeutic action to wrap the affected part with a cloth, previous friction with plantain soaked in oil. It is a traditional Basque remedy.

To relieve bruises

Apply to the affected limb very hot or almost boiling salt water.

Against bone fractures

A first cure is to cover the fractured limb with a poultice of wheat flour bran, eggs and wine. Then, put the patient in the hands of a healer or a doctor.

To remove thorns stuck in the limb

Place on the affected area pork gall.

If a hawthorn thorn is stuck in the wound

To heal the wound produced by the hawthorn barb, the affected person must ask for forgiveness from the bush.

***

But perhaps it is better to do the same as before: put some pork gall to soften the skin, open the pore and remove the thorn.

Against burns

Put lye quickly on the burned area.

Put on toothpaste.

***

Cut slices of new potato and apply on the burn. In addition to relieving the pain, this will prevent blisters from developing.

***

Applying salt or bicarbonate to the lesion can have a similar effect.

***

Cut garlic in quantity, crush well, add oil and put it all in a poultice on the burned part.

***

Take a handful of garlic cloves, crush them, put them to boil and when they are boiling, remove the oil and add virgin wax. Make a paste and put it on the burn.

***

If you have nothing better at hand, smear the affected area with oil, preferably olive oil.

***

Keep the injured area near the fire as long as possible so that blisters do not appear. The same is achieved by applying cow dung to the burn. Then cover with unsalted butter and bandage.

***

Collect snow in a bottle and keep it tightly closed. Apply this water to the burns when necessary.

***

If the sun has been too much on the head and has produced sunstroke, place a small glass of water upside down on a cloth and press on the head until the water absorbs the heat.

***

Or immerse the feet in a basin of very hot water mixed with ash and bran. It is also an excellent remedy against painful menstruation.

***

If the burn has produced milk, oil or boiling water, paint the lesions with black ink using a brush.

Against sunburns

Crush a tomato and mix with two tablespoons of baking soda. Spread on the burned skin and let stand for half an hour.

***

Similar results can be obtained with melon juice mixed with olive oil.

***

Rub the burned areas with vinegar, but do not rub too hard.

Against frostbite

When a limb suffers from symptoms of frostbite, soak it in water to which burning embers have been poured beforehand.

***

Water with salt and red bell pepper are also useful.

Against cramps

Wet the affected person with saliva on the index finger of the right hand, draw with it a cross on the attacked part and rub it afterwards.

***

Rub the affected area with rosemary water or cow marrow.

***

According to a Galician remedy, cramps disappear if they are blessed three times with an old sickle, on the edge of which a few drops have been spilled.

According to a Galician remedy, cramps disappear if they are blessed three times with an old sickle, on whose edge a few drops of blood of snake, mixed with bat blood, have been spilled.

***

If the cramp occurs in a leg, step on something cold barefoot.

***

To avoid cramps, walk on your back for a while.

***

A Castilian remedy to avoid the annoying cramp consisted in placing a bar of homemade soap between the mattress and the sheets of the person who feared suffering from it.

***

Place a magnet at the bottom of the bed of the sufferer, with the tips pointing towards the feet of the sufferer.

To remove a nailed splinter

To heal a wound caused by splinters or remove a splinter, put snakeskin smeared with oil on the area.

To heal bruises

Rub the bruised area with absorbent cotton soaked in wine, oil and sugar, previously beaten together.

***

Boil water with salt and apply it to the bruised area with a strong message.

To soften the abscesses

Those annoying abscesses that appear on the extremities of the fingers heal very well. For example, they are softened by soaking them in bread soaked in milk.

***

Spread garlic on the abscess or rub a lemon peel on the abscess.

***

Burn an onion, pour oil on it and rub the painful area of inflammation with it.

***

Put bay leaves on the abscess, three if possible.

***

It is better if, while they are placed on the affected area, the area is sanctified with each bay leaf while the patient prays a Creed.

***

Put the sick finger in pork gall, previously put to temper.

***

Make a poultice with wine, oil, lard, linseed, garlic, onion and rennet. Put it all over the toe.

***

But surely this is the most traditional remedy of all: pour water into a pot, then pour the water into a pot when it is already warm. Inside the pot, place the pot face down and on top of it a comb; on top of it, two laurel branches in the shape of a cross, and on top of that, a pair of open scissors, also in the shape of a cross. On top of all this, put your finger on the panadizo.

Against drowning

If someone is about to die from drowning, place his head down and apply hot plasters on his chest.

CANCER

Although with all the qualms in the world, some remedies against different types of cancer are collected here, which, surprisingly, gave positive results. This does not mean that it is convenient to try them without further ado, but it is true that hope, especially when official medicine fails or does not arrive, is the last thing that should be lost.

Against skin cancer

Official medicine today seems to be able to offer some hope for a solution to this disease. However, until about twenty years ago, it was apparently cured by a Canary Island healer from La Palma, according to the following remedy, which she kept secret as long as she lived: prepare an ointment with arsenic paste and bee honey. Apply the paste to the lesion and leave it on for twenty-four hours. Then wash with mallow water, and repeat the operation every eight days. Then prepare an ointment with virgin wax, balsam and olive oil, which should be cooked until it is thick. Place it on the wound as a poultice, repeating the operation twice a day until the scab is lifted. If the wound is particularly stubborn, heat the ointment in a limpet shell and apply it to the wound. Repeat the cycle every eight days until the wound is healed.

Against a localized cancerous tumor

If you have a localized and open cancerous tumor, place a piece of fresh meat on the affected area daily. Apparently, placing a live toad that eats the diseased part in the wound still gives better results.

***

If you have a tumor in a limb and want to know if it is benign or not, get a wooden container, one of those used to sell herring, and make several holes in its base. Enclose two toads inside and cover the container, which will then be placed on the damaged part, fastened with a bandage. The patient will be healed if the toads are still alive the next day, not so if the animals appear dead.

THE WOMAN'S PROBLEMS

Here we will say no more: For a good future, it is necessary to give birth safely.

For a trouble-free menstruation

If menstruations are irregular or painful, take infusions of parsley root, but outside of meals.

***

Or infusions of worm herb, also called tansy (Tanacetum vulgare).

***

If the period is delayed, take two daily infusions, outside meals, of sea fennel (Crithmum maritimum).

***

Mugwort oil has also been used to regulate menstrual cycles.

***

Many women are in the habit of bandaging an ankle during menstruation, believing that during this period, the bones are weakened, with the consequent risk of sprains.

To alleviate the problems of menopause

Take infusions of white dictamo, also known as fresnillo (Dictamnus albus), when hot flashes occur.

***

Eat products abundant in calcium to strengthen the bones. It is a popular belief that during this critical period of a woman's life, her skeleton weakens, and she is more prone to suffer bone fractures, especially hip fractures.

***

Follow a diet based on fresh vegetables, combined with some physical exercise.

Against some problems of the female parts

Against uterine haemorrhages, insert into the vagina pieces of sour lemon, cut in half, and plug the vulva with gauze. Tie the thighs with bandages to facilitate greater external pressure.

***

Against vaginal infections, wash the female parts with oak leaves and oak bark decoctions.

***

If the infected is the vaginal discharge, take the infusion resulting from cooking five or seven-bay leaves in a quart of water.

***

Soak with a decoction of oak to prevent inflammation caused by uterine prolapse. The best part is the webbing between the bark and trunk or under the acorn husk.

To promote fertility

This is an ancient remedy against sterility: Drink on an empty stomach, the woman who can not have children, a tablespoon of sage juice with a little salt for nine consecutive days. The second night, roast a fresh egg that is soft and break it with the weight of a timin or pinch of ground lupin (Lavandula latifolia), and stir it all as if it were salt, eat it when you go to sleep, but not before taking a little carrot seed with good wine. Do not take chocolate during the treatment.

***

Another somewhat more brutal remedy, corresponding to the tradition, recommended giving the woman hare's rennet dissolved in hot water; if she had pains, she was fit to procreate.

***

And more curious, is the remedy consisting of placing on the bed of the infertile woman some pants belonging to a man of proven fertility, better if it is done on the night of San Juan.

***

In order to remain in a state of good hope, many French women have tried a formula consisting of wearing their husband's shirt and pants for a season.

Abortions

The parsley introduced in the vagina is abortive. In some places, they have used a cane to make it reach the neck of the uterus.

***

Although of lesser effect, it has been to apply on the navel of the pregnant woman a poultice of parsley crushed with garlic.

***

The infusions of ergot are also abortive, as well as the decoctions of buckthorn berries, cursed roses or peony, carrot grana, foxglove and the drinks resulting from boiling various herbs.

***

The immoderate ingestion of female broccoli decoctions has traditionally been considered abortive and highly toxic. For this reason, and in spite of the popular use it has been given, its consumption is not recommended.

***

The ingestion of díctamo root bark decoction, also known as Fresnillo, can also provoke an abortion in pregnant women.

***

Some components of rue are very abortive and very dangerous, to the point of having caused many deaths of pregnant women.

And the ingestion of celery.

***

And the decoctions of yarrow, so they are not recommended during pregnancy.

***

On the contrary, to avoid miscarriage, some pregnant women have taken infusions of bistort (Polygonum bistorta).

Aids for pregnant women

To be successful, the pregnant woman should abstain from eating herbs such as rue, parsley and ergot, which are abortifacients.

***

Take lots of fruit and infusions of linden blossom before going to bed.

***

To give strength to the parturient, take the interesting infusions of hyssop (Hyssopus officinalis).

***

If the parturient has very dry or narrow secretory parts, or her belly is very sensitive to the touch, it is necessary to apply sitz baths. For this, there is nothing better than for her to receive the vapours resulting from the decoction of a handful of flax seeds or marshmallow root, with the vulva immersed in the liquid itself. It is better if the Boiled is composed of mallow, marshmallow, Parietaria, mercurial and mullein, and even better, all administered in doses of a handful.

To facilitate childbirth

There is no natural remedy that works. The best thing to do is to call an expert midwife or to take the pregnant woman, when it is time to give birth, to the doctor or, better still, to a qualified midwife. Anything else would be a dangerous gamble with the health of the woman and her unborn child. However, let us know a few remedies, all of them pilgrimish and already out of use, or which should be out of use for the good of future mothers.

***

If labor is particularly difficult or complicated, apply fresh horse manure, cooked in vinegar or spider webs, to the vulva and vagina of the parturient. Although it sounds like a joke, this remedy was used by a prestigious doctor of the sixteenth century, no less than with an empress, but without success ... because the sick woman died.

***

When the contractions begin, blow on the belly of the parturient.

***

Provoke her nausea by putting a hare's ear in her mouth, biting her own braid of hair or drinking her husband's urine.

***

To give her strength in the trance of childbirth, bite the parturient a stick between her teeth or blow through a bottle.

***

Or give her a rubbing with a red muleteer's cloth.

***

It also helps to give birth well to tie to the waist of the parturient the end of the rope of a church bell, which will ring three times.

***

All these remedies will be reinforced if a piece of iron is placed on the bed of the parturient.

***

It has been believed that to facilitate the expulsion of the child, it was convenient to step with the foot on the parturient's stomach and press with the fists on her kidneys.

***

It was a widespread belief in half of Europe that it helps to give birth if the woman has at the moment of delivery some male garment on her body, preferably of her husband or the father of the child. For such a purpose, they have been used, especially some pants of the spouse, which have been extended on the body of the parturient. Some, taking their propitiatory precautions further, have considered it essential to pass these pants nine times over the body of the parturient, with the legs upwards, then to take them to the door of the house and to strike them nine times. After being beaten, even more, the pants in question are finally burned in some areas.

***

In some areas of Extremadura, the oldest and most worn male hat has been put on her during childbirth to make childbirth easier for a woman.

***

To prevent the child from breeching, the mother's waist is wrapped with a silk ribbon, knotted at the back.

***

If the baby is pierced, let the parturient drink milk from another woman's breast.

***

If labor is delayed, place two crossed ash sticks on the belly of the parturient.

***

Or peel and crush lily root, mix it with virgin honey and introduce it into the vagina of the parturient.

To expel the placenta

To facilitate the expulsion of the placenta, take a decoction of hazel mistletoe.

***

Irrigate the woman's parts with an infusion of mallows.

***

Bite the newly delivered woman a lock of her own hair.

***

Drink the milk of another woman mixed with oil.

Or drink ground jet mixed with wine.

Against infections of the womb

Remedy that under no circumstances should be put into practice consisted in the past if an infection was seen in the womb of the woman who had just given birth, to gather all the other women in the house and make them urinate in a container. Vaginal irrigation was practised on the sick woman with a mixture of all the urine.

***

So that no problem affects the puérpera, after childbirth, the first clothes the parturient wears are smoked with green laurel and grains of wheat.

***

When the womb hurts after childbirth, apply to the patient; in the lower abdomen, a poultice of rue is crushed with two cloves of garlic.

***

To mitigate the pains that childbirth can produce, smoke the private parts of the parturient by burning partridge or chicken feathers. The remedy also serves to cut the haemorrhages of the womb.

To breastfeed well

In some Central European countries, such as Poland, Slovakia and the Czech Republic, new mothers have been drinking beer moderately, at lunch and dinner, to gain teat and quantity of milk. In modern times, this custom has been extended to much more southern European areas and has even leaped America.

***

The newborn baby should drink chicken broth during the three days following the birth to avoid the fevers that solid food can cause.

***

Drink plenty of orange and pure lemon juice to avoid possible infections.

***

Eat garlic and onion in large quantities, for example, with a salad of lettuce, tomato and boiled potatoes.

***

To gain in milk, take green fennel leaves cooked with wine.

***

Or drink infusions of the fruit of dill, crushed and pulverized.

To remove the milk

When the baby is well breastfed and can eat other things, but the woman still has milk coming out, in order to remove it, drink parsley root water.

***

Let the mother drink infusion of cane, taking parsley under the sole of the foot, inside the shoes.

***

Drink celery infusions.

***

Also, the ingestion of sage has served to remove milk from women, but its use proved more dangerous than beneficial.

***

Put hot cabbage leaves on the woman's back.

***

Put cabbage leaves, smeared with unsalted butter, on the woman's back; on them, put well-chopped parsley, and two cabbage leaves on the breasts. The milk will stop in one day.

***

Place on the breasts of the mother, wrapped in a handkerchief, garlic in handfuls, well crushed and with salt.

***

Rub the woman's breasts with hen's butter, but without salt.

***

Another remedy, as traditional as it is ancient, consists of the woman breastfeeding the children of other females who have not had milk.

***

In the past, in many villages, women gave their milk to beggars or to orphaned fools.

***

Or they would put a puppy dog on the teat, so it would suckle directly from her.

***

In some places, the custom of lactating women was to milk their breasts over the fire or in the water of a stream.

***

If, in spite of everything, the little one persists in suckling, the mother should apply bitter or spicy products on the nipple, and the baby will not take long to reject them.

Against sores and cracks on the nipples

Apply sugar and lard plasters.

Or plasters of crushed partridge's feet.

***

Apply on the breasts cloths soaked in water where berries from the cypress trees of the village cemetery have been boiled.

***

Rub the affected breasts daily with slices of lemon with salt.

***

Wash the breasts of women with sores on the nipples daily with brandy.

Against hardening of the breasts

Apply on the breasts of the interested woman a dressing of thread cloth, impregnated in the paste resulting from frying in pure olive oil, the following products: virgin wax, honey, brandy, chopped black tobacco, hen's milk, olive twigs and a laurel leaf blessed on Palm Sunday.

***

Prepare nine bundles with three kinds of herbs: fennel, cattail and wormwood (although others can be added). Follow the hardened area of the chest with each of the bunches, from top to bottom and from left to right. Recite at the same time the following formula: "Zingiri sor † blood † Zingiri Salomon. I do not sign you except by the grace of the Holy Spirit". Sanctify the healer at the same time, nine times, dipping the hand in holy water, one each time. Once the operation is finished, recite nine Our Fathers and burn the herbs in a pot, applying the incineration smoke to the patient's chest. If the pain does not subside on the first day, repeat the ensalmos on the second day. If the pain does not disappear despite it, abandon the procedure because it will no longer work. It was a typical remedy of some Basque healers.

***

Make crosses with a rosary on the breasts of the patient.

***

According to a Portuguese remedy, rub the breasts of the affected woman with the husband's shirt. It will be even more effective if the sufferer of mammary inflammation sleeps with her husband's panties across the bed.

***

145

Mastitis in its first stage is prevented by rubbing the patient's breasts with unsalted chicken lard. You can also place on the breasts, wrapped in a handkerchief, which must be white, with well-crushed garlic and salt.

Care for the newborn

First, always keep him/her clean.

***

Against procedures, talcum powder. Use wood powder if there is no such, which is already difficult in any place, no matter how remote.

***

It is very good for the baby's skin. The powder results from squeezing roasted oregano between the fingers.

***

Rub the sores that may come out of the child with egg white beaten in water.

***

Also, use beaten oil, also in water, for the same purpose.

***

For constipation, insert a stalk of cabbage rubbed in oil, or parsley, also rubbed in oil, into the anus of the infant.

***

When the child starts teething and his gums hurt, rub him gently with a thimble or a sugar cube.

***

This was a common remedy until very recently to make the holes in the ears of girls heal well when putting earrings in them: Lean the ear lobe on a potato and prick the lobe with a threaded needle thread to be left in the hole. To facilitate healing, smear saliva on daily fasting and move the thread to form the hole.

Against the alferecía

If it is a newborn baby, this disease is avoided by giving it to drink a drop of water in a container, bowl or silver instrument.

***

To cure it, prepare some powders with the three entrails of a hedgehog -these are the liver, the lungs and the heart in the following way: With a very sharp knife, open the back of the hedgehog while it is still alive, and before it cools, tear out with your hands the said entrails, taking care not to separate them from the diaphragm or the gall. Hang such entrails in a dry and ventilated place until, well cured, they can be ground. Of course, apart from its curative effectiveness, this product will not be pleasant to the palate.

FINAL NOTE

Here ends this small contribution to the popular medicine, but it ends only halfway because it is formally promised the digital edition, soon, of a second instalment dedicated to that more intimate, secret and problematic part of the human body, which has to do with the perpetuation of the human species, and to everything that from the point of view of the folkloric tradition -home remedies, superstitions, magic, etc.- is related to it.

But, before ending this book, or to end it as you prefer, and although it may seem rude to some, this author cannot resist saying goodbye without including a well-known saying in rural areas, which comes to express in a clear way what health means for popular thought, and which, in short, concludes that everyone is the best healer of himself: Piss clear, pee dry and shit hard... and send the doctor to hell.

José Dueso, December 2013

MINIMAL BIBLIOGRAPHY

In addition to the information obtained by word of mouth, which is essential for preparing this work, we have consulted numerous books, articles and even handwritten notes from many different sources. As some of them are of great antiquity and are not available to the general public, we will mention only the most accessible ones so as not to make this report too long.

Analysis of the popular Basque medicine. Anton Erkoreka. Labayru Institute. Bilbao, 1985.

Ancient popular medicine. R. Benito Vidal. Abraxas Editions. Barcelona, 1998.

Apellaniz. Past and present of a village in Alava. Gerardo López de Gereñu. In Estudios de Etnografía alavesa. OHITURA, nº 2. Provincial Council of Alava. Vitoria-Gasteiz, 1981.

Aproximación a la folkmedicina de Cartagena. Carlos Fernández Araujo. NARRIA, nº 49-50. Madrid, 1988.

Notes on the life of Lagrán. Salustiano Viana. In Estudios de Etnografía alavesa. O HITURA, nº 2. Provincial Council of Alava. Vitoria-Gasteiz, 1984.

Brujería y otros oficios populares de la magia (Witchcraft and other popular magic crafts). Juan Francisco Blanco. Ambito Ediciones. Valladolid, 1992. Brujology. San Sebastian Congress. Papers and Communications. Seminarios y Ediciones. Madrid, 1975. Marriage in Aragón, El. Rafael Andolz. General Bookstore. Zaragoza, 1993.

Chapters of Basque folk medicine. Ángel Goicoetxea Marcaida. University of Salamanca, 1983.

Shamanism in the Amazon, El. Carlos Junquera. Editorial Mitre. Barcelona, n. d.

Lost "Kitchen", The. Josep María Gorrís. Queimada Ediciones. Barcelona, 1980.

Sexual behavior of the Basques. José María Satrústegui. Editorial Txertoa. Donostia-San Sebastián, 1981.

Contribution to the ethnographic study of the continental Basque Country. Juan Thalamus. In Anuario de Eusko-Folklore, XI. Vitoria-Gasteiz, 1931.

Costumari català. Joan Amades. Salvat Ediciones. Barcelona, 1986. Aragonese customs. Antonio Beltrán. Editorial Everest. León, 1990. Asturian customs. Elvira Martínez. Editorial Everest. León, 1986.

Canarian customs, traditions and medicinal remedies. José Luis Concepción. Editorial José Luis Concepción. La Laguna, 1993.

Body in the traditional society, El. Françoise Loux. Olañeta Editor. Palma de Mallorca, 1984.

Data for a study of folk medicine in Goizueta. J. Ormazabal. In Anuario de Eusko-Folklore, XXV. Vitoria-Gasteiz, 1973-74.

Dictionary of demonology. Frederik Koning. Editorial Bruguera. Barcelona, 1975.

Dictionary of medicinal plants. Óscar Yarza. Distribuciones Mateo. Madrid, 1984.

Where, how, and when to collect medicinal plants. Eugenio G. Vaga. Editorial De Vecchi. Barcelona, 1981.

Cutaneous diseases in the popular Basque medicine, Las. Ángel Goicoetxea Marcaida. Notebooks of the History of Basque Medicine. Monographs, No. 1. Salamanca, 1981.

Ethnography of Reus and its region. El Camp, la Conca de Barberà, el Priorat. Ramon Violant i Simorra. Editorial Alta Fulla. Barcelona, 1990.

Popular ethnomedicine. Ángel Carril. Castilla Ediciones. Valladolid, 1991.

Galician folklore. Emilia Pardo Bazán and others. Roger Editor. Donostia-San Sebastián, 2000.

Galicia: witchcraft, superstition and mysticism. Ana Liste. Penthalon Editions. Madrid, 1981.

Gran libro de las supersticiones, El. Peter Lorie. Robinbook Editions. Barcelona, 1993.

Guía del curanderismo en España y disciplinas paralelas. Jaume Vicens Carrió. Martínez Roca Editions. Barcelona, 1985.

Herbs that heal. Edmund Chessi and B. Pozas Hermosilla. Barcelona, 1985.

History of medicine. Albert S. Lyons and Joseph Petrucelli. Doyma Ediciones. Barcelona, 1984.

Manual de folklore. La vida popular tradicional en España. Luis de Hoyos Sainz and Nieves de Hoyos Sancho. Istmo Editions. Madrid, 1985.

Medicina en el Camino de Santiago, La. Luis de Campo. Príncipe de Viana, XXVII. Iruñea-Pamplona, 1966.

Medicina, malaltia i salut a Catalunya. Josep Maria Comelles. In Traditions and legends, vol. Edicions Mateu. Barcelona, 1982.

Medicina popular. Joan Amades. In Arxiu de tradicions populars, fascicle III. Barcelona, 1928.

Medicina popular. José Dueso. Volume IV of Nosotros los vascos. Myths, beliefs and customs. Editorial Lur. Donostia-San Sebastián, 1989.

Popular medicine. Arantzazu Hurtado de Saracho. Iruñea-Pamplona. 1976.

Medicina popular, La. Montserrat Puigdengolas and Regina Miranda. Editorial DOPESA. Barcelona, 1978. Medicina popular en el País Vasco, La. Ignacio María Barriola. Basque Editions. Donostia-San Sebastián, 1979. Medicina popular en el País Vasco, La. José María Satrústegui. Gaceta Médica de Bilbao, No. 73. Bilbao, 1976 Medicina popular en España. Ingrid Kuschick. Siglo Veintiuno de España Editores. Madrid, 1995.

Medicina popular interpretada, La. Xosé Ramón Mariño Ferro. Edicións Xerais de Galicia. Santiago de Compostela, 1985.

Medicina popular y primera infancia. José María Satrústegui. Cuadernos de Etnología y Etnografía, No. 30. Prince of Viana Foundation. Iruñea-Pamplona, 1978.

Basque folk medicine and gynecology. José María Satrústegui. Cuadernos de Etnología y Etnografía, No. 27. Fundación Príncipe de Viana. Iruñea-Pamplona, 1977.

Valencian magic and popular medicine. Juan Gil Barberá and Enric Martí Mora. Carena Editors. Valencia, 1997.

Mythology and superstitions of Cantabria. Adriano García-Lomas. Estvdio Bookstore. Santander, 2000.

Other medicines, The. Florence Arnold-Richez. Ediciones Parramón Ediciones. Barcelona, 1983.

Small guide to medicinal plants. Elfrune Wendelberg. Barcelona, 1981. Spanish Pyrenees, The. Ramon Violant i Simorra. Editorial Altafulla. Barcelona, 1989. Medicinal plants. Margarita Fernández and Ana Nieto. Iruñea-Pamplona, 1982.

Medicinal plants. Pío Font Quer. Editorial Labor. Barcelona, 1990.

Medicinal plants. Revista Mundo Científico, no. 105. September, 1990.

Plantas silvestres y cultivadas en la gastronomía común, vegetariana y medicinal, Las. Juan Mugarza. Bilbao, 1988.

Rama dorada, La. J. G. Frazer. Fondo de Cultura Económico. Madrid, 1986.

Recetas y remedios en la medicina popular vasca. José Miguel de Barandiarán. Editorial Txertoa. Donostia-San Sebastián, 1989.

Remeis casolans. David Griñó i Garriga (L'Herbolari de la Riera del Pi). Editorial Millà. Barcelona, 1976.

Rite and formula in Basque folk medicine. Health through medicinal plants. Juan Garmendia Larrañaga. Editorial Txertoa. Donostia-San Sebastián, 1980.

Superstitions from Extremadura. Publio Hurtado. Edited by Alfonso Artero Hurtado. Huelva, 1989.

Superstitions and beliefs of Asturias. Luciano Castañón. Ayalga Ediciones. Salinas, 1982.

Daily life in Muslim Spain, La. Fernando Díaz-Plaja. Editorial Edaf. Madrid, 1993.

Made in the USA
Monee, IL
26 November 2024

71344437R00089